THE PRE-PREGNANCY PLANNER

THE
PRE-PREGNANCY
PLANNER

JOSLEEN WILSON

Introduction by
Joseph H. Bellina, M.D., PH.D.

DOUBLEDAY & COMPANY, INC.
GARDEN CITY, NEW YORK
1986

Please note that we have changed the names of all the people who were
kind enough to let me interview them in order to protect their privacy.

Library of Congress Cataloging-in-Publication Data
Wilson, Josleen.
The pre-pregnancy planner.

Includes index.
1. Pregnancy—Planning.   I. Title.
RG525.F454   1986   618.2'4   85-30737
ISBN 9780385231749

146718297

CONTENTS

CONTENTS   ix

INTRODUCTION

FOR MOST WOMEN, going through pregnancy and childbirth will be the most physically and mentally grueling experience in their lives. It is amazing to me that while athletes routinely spend months and even years building up endurance and preparing their bodies and minds for competition, the majority of women are woefully underprepared for the greatest marathon they will ever run: having a baby. *The Pre-Pregnancy Planner* is the training manual these future expectant mothers so desperately need.

Almost every person who thinks about starting a family today is faced with staggering obstacles: emotional ambivalence, money problems, inadequate living space, uncertain marriages, career complications, concern for children from previous marriages. On top of this are health issues never dreamed of twenty years ago—infertility, environmental toxins, alcohol, smoking, and drugs.

In the past decade we doctors have acquired much new scientific information about pregnancy and its outcome. Today with technological developments we can tell within three days of conception that a pregnancy is developing; using ultrasound scans we can accurately guess the sex of the child and determine many birth defects; with other tests such as amniocentesis we can determine blood type, birth defects due to chromosome abnormalities, and other hereditary diseases.

But the one thing the medical profession has not addressed is the need for a systematic preparation *before* pregnancy—and every day we are learning just how valuable such preparation is to future parents and their offspring.

In terms of health, numerous studies have shown that problems such as miscarriage, birth defects, and underweight newborns, as well as problems for children later in life, may have been caused not by what the mother did while she was pregnant but what she did beforehand. Even fathers come in for their share of the blame. Every woman preparing for motherhood is a product of her total ecology system—not only her reproductive organs, but her overall physical condition, her diet, her emotional outlook, and the environment in which she lives. *The Pre-Pregnancy Planner* places all of these systems together in a logical order so that prospective parents can deal with each vital issue adequately *before* conception.

In addition to the body of current knowledge brought together here, *The Pre-Pregnancy Planner* introduces new information about diet and exercise imperative for women contemplating pregnancy.

The nine months of pregnancy once adequate for incorporating a baby into marriage is no longer enough time to grapple with the many emotional, work-related, and financial concerns of parenthood in modern society. Today the physical reality of pregnancy may actually be too late to make certain decisions about how a child will fit into the scheme of things in a healthy and enjoyable way.

At the Omega Institutes, where we specialize in working with infertile couples, I've met many couples whose most treasured goal is for the wife to become pregnant and have a baby. They are often so caught up with the quest for pregnancy that they fail to consider how their lives will change after the child is born. They haven't really figured out how to take care of the child, nor have they coped with financial issues and career adjustments. It's as if childbirth is the only goal, and the baby will always be a few weeks old. They do not project the child's future across even the next five years. When the baby arrives they are overwhelmed with problems they never dreamed of and this reality turns parenting into a chaotic, stressful experience, instead of the blissful rapture they had anticipated.

In the same vein, many people prepared to spend several thousand dollars to achieve a first-class childbirth experience think that once the child arrives, the expense miraculously disappears and that three can live for the same price as two. The initial cost is probably the least expensive part of having a child. In my own personal experience of raising two boys who are now grown up, I can testify that there are expenses that one would never dream of that consistently crop up. With children, the unusual expense becomes the ordinary, everyday occurrence. Today even couples who are certain their incomes would never warrant consulting a financial planner should consider making long-term financial plans for their children.

In short, there are many factors that have to be considered beyond the simple fact of pregnancy itself. *The Pre-Pregnancy Planner* gives a realistic approach to what a child means in the life of a couple—in terms of emotions, finances, careers, and health. So don't wait until you're pregnant to read this book.

The Pre-Pregnancy Planner is divided into four sections.

"Making a Decision" helps women and men resolve emotional conflicts by explaining how having a baby affects existing family relationships, career and financial planning, and it anticipates ways to cope with child care. The growing complexity of modern life, of changing male and female roles, of shifting family structures means that childbirth is no longer an automatic goal of marriage. This section spells out the emotional realities of what it means to be a parent today, so that decisions can be made thoughtfully and maturely before conception instead of afterward, when it may be too late.

"Health and Fitness for Pregnancy" shows what every woman considering pregnancy can do for herself and her baby by taking into account her nutrition and physical fitness. And I mean *every* woman contemplating pregnancy—regardless of her age or current health.

A child's prenatal environment is a direct reflection of the parents' environment. New environmental menaces face the modern woman —job hazards, pollution, exposure from low-dose X rays, smoking, drugs, food additives, chemicals, alcohol—and all can have an impact on the child's future health. This section contains the latest scientific information on environmental hazards that might endanger your baby even before you become pregnant. It is a detox program, highlighted by the first diet ever devised to prepare the modern woman for pregnancy, as well as a special exercise shape-up that concentrates on those areas of the body placed under most stress during pregnancy. A vital Pre-Pregnancy Checklist, which lists the issues to pay attention to before pregnancy and describes a medical exam for women thinking about becoming pregnant, rounds out this section.

Section Three, "Special Pre-Pregnancy Considerations," elaborates on exciting new scientific developments that can affect your plans for parenting: when genetic counseling is a must, preparing for high-risk pregnancies, helping older women becoming mothers, coping with miscarriage, inroads into infertility, and new fertility technologies.

The final section of the book, "Ready for Pregnancy," answers practical questions about the early weeks of pregnancy. What can you expect in the way of maternity care in America today? How, and when, should you choose an obstetrician and hospital? What will happen when you first become pregnant, and what adjustments can you plan to make in your life?

The Pre-Pregnancy Planner gives planned parenthood a whole new meaning. In my opinion this book forecasts a new field of study for physicians and scientists, as well as for prospective parents. It will be a tremendous resource for anyone thinking of having a child. I feel certain that pre-pregnancy planning will become a standard procedure as more and more prospective parents become aware of the need to think, explore, and plan before they conceive. The widespread adoption of pre-pregnancy planning may well be the best news in years for the families of the future.

A child does not ask to be born. A child is the product of two people who decide that they will produce a third person. The child has no control over the process. It's the responsibility of the parents to give that child the best that life in their world has to offer.

If you are planning to become pregnant, preparing yourself properly—getting your body in shape, working out the details of careers and finances, making plans for good medical care—means that you can be relaxed and positive about the future. Good preparation is rewarding physically and emotionally, and it can make pregnancy and childbirth a pleasure.

A few hours of reading *The Pre-Pregnancy Planner* can make the difference between a family faced with doubts and anxieties, and a family looking forward to a healthy, happy parenting experience.

January 1986

—JOSEPH H. BELLINA, M.D., PH.D.
National Advisor to the Child and Human Development Council of the National Institutes of Health, and Director of the Omega Institutes, a New Orleans-based women's hospital specializing in infertility

THE PRE-PREGNANCY PLANNER

PART ONE

MAKING
A DECISION

CHAPTER 1

CHOOSING PARENTHOOD

PEOPLE ONCE TOOK IT for granted that they would marry and have children. But women and men are more thoughtful about parenthood today, less certain about the futures their children will inherit, more concerned with their own places in the world, as a couple and as individuals. Because American society is more complex than it has ever been, it's not surprising that many approach parenthood with many reservations and some trepidation.

Childbirth has always been subject to various social mandates, but having a baby today is vulnerable to an inordinate number of trends. Options about the timing of marriage and children abound. A variety of family styles—dual-career, blended, single-parent, communal—flourish.

Nor are relationships the simple boy-meets-girl-and-gets-married mechanism of the past. New reports published by the Census Bureau point out that the number of unmarried men and women living together has more than tripled since 1970, climbing to nearly two million couples. When live-in couples make the commitment to marry it is often because they have decided to have a baby. When the marriage decision is tied up with the baby decision, couples face the changes that marital commitment inevitably brings at the same time that they face the changes of parenthood.

Some single women who have postponed marriage fear that they will run into a biological wall and are deciding to bear children without partners. Once an extremely rare occurrence, some two hundred thousand single American women have chosen to become pregnant, often via artificial insemination, in the last five years.

These original social trends mean that there is more latitude than ever before in terms of if and when to marry, and if and when to have children. At the same time, actually making the decision is more complicated than ever. Freedom to choose has brought its burdens.

Even Dr. Benjamin Spock, that eminent proponent of parenthood, has written, "No woman could have a totally positive attitude toward an event that permanently changes the course of her life as much as pregnancy does."

Pregnancy means growth; with birth comes change. And both processes can bring conflict. "Ambivalence—not just about pregnancy, but about everything—is the natural human condition," says noted psychoanalyst and author Janet Jeppson. "There is no one way to make a decision about parenthood, and each person has to work out his or her own scheme."

A BABY: YES OR NO?

Implicit in the promise of modern birth control is the idea that couples can decide not only when, but *if,* they would have children. Birth control and other changes in modern society have made the choice to remain child-free a legitimate option.

Men and women are asking themselves, "Will I be a good parent? Can I rear a happy child? Can I be a better parent than my mother and father?" In a society where both partners work to make ends meet, couples face financial obstacles unique in our time. Women who have professional careers may ask themselves if they are trying to prove that they are superwomen by also having children. Society, with its constantly changing trends, mores, and economic fluctuations, pushes the individual first along one path, then another.

When a couple like Jeannette and Lawrence, with a good marriage and two well-paying jobs, decide against parenthood, "society" calls them selfish. "All they care about is themselves," may be a running comment in their families. A woman who rejects motherhood is typically said to have "missed out." "She's not a real woman." Men, too, are likely to have their virility measured by offspring.

When surrounded by an emphatic chorus of thumbs up or thumbs down, it's hard for a man or woman to make a personal choice. The mental health community further complicates the decision-making process. Most therapists still hold that having children is a strong, natural human instinct and not having babies is deviant.

In spite of many prejudices, some singular voices have suggested that childbearing today is not a societal obligation, but a personal choice. Family therapist Sonya Rhodes, co-author of *Surviving Family Life,* believes that "the choice to remain child-free is neither more nor less healthy than the choice to have a family. But making a rational decision means being able to consider both possibilities objectively."

A Man's Decision, Too

According to Dr. Rhodes, the decision to have a baby is a genuine choice that a couple should share. Nevertheless, women are seen as the force behind parenthood, with men going along because it's expected of them. In some ways, men have even less room than women to reject parenthood, and many hesitate to even admit their anxieties about fatherhood.

It Takes Two

Readiness to bear children does not always come to both partners at the same time. Differences in desire can make the decision more difficult.

Desire for children is often out of sync when partners are of different ages, or at different stages of their personal development. A younger woman married to an older husband, for example, may not want to produce instant babies just so he can avoid "being a grandfather" to his children. An older husband, already supporting teenagers from a previous marriage, may feel anxious about his second wife's yearning for children of her own.

Further, what two people agreed on before marriage, if they discussed children, may not be what they agree on after two or five years of married life. Even within good marriages, arguments occur over the number and timing of children.

Each partner's individual style of decision making may prolong ambivalence. Some people make decisions strictly on an intellectual level; others lean toward intuitiveness. Some believe in going with the flow. (Oddly, for many people, the bigger the decision, the more likely they are to leave it to chance.) In trying to make a decision about babies, couples can spend most of their time arguing about whose "style" is correct—emotional or intellectual.

In general, couples who are happily married have worked out ways of matching their styles and making decisions that take into account each person's feelings. But it can be frustrating when one person wants children and his or her partner doesn't—at least not yet. If one of you is worried about finances or jobs, the other must take these concerns seriously. It may be necessary to talk these issues through with an impartial third party, such as a marriage counselor.

Deciding Not to Decide

Many people still prefer to avoid, at least overtly, making a choice. Some simply postpone making a decision, and others would rather take life as it comes.

Most of the young couples I talked with use some method of birth control, anticipating the time when they will feel secure enough to start adding new lives to their households. And frequently their "accidental" pregnancies are unconsciously planned.

Jill Ferguson believes in a simple approach. "If everyone had to go through all that agonizing before having a child, they'd never do it. In my case, we had been married three years, when I accidentally got pregnant. We were both working, and while we weren't rich by any means, we were okay. And I was thirty-three years old. Well, we said, why not? But if I had to consciously decide, I'd still be lying on the beach in East Hampton."

An accidental pregnancy is not necessarily an unwanted one. It depends on the circumstances surrounding the birth, as well as on the adaptability of the parents. Some couples take it philosophically, recognizing that there really is no completely convenient time to have a baby. The number of children already in the family and the space between them are two important factors. If there is a basic fault in the marital relationship, however, the pressures of an accidental pregnancy are likely to bring it into the open.

Resolving Ambivalence

Even when we *do* wish to make a conscious decision, we can still be paralyzed by the notion. Although making a decision is completely personal and individual—to a great extent each person has to figure it out on his or her own—professional counselors have gathered some guidelines to help couples analyze their readiness for pregnancy.

Debra Gajer, a social worker for the Margaret Sanger Center of Planned Parenthood in New York City, who works with people debating parenthood, says that finances are the biggest concern for prospective parents today. The major problem: loss or reduction of the woman's income. Career and educational objectives and plans for the future are also major worries.

Gajer counsels couples to sit down together and talk about their fears and insecurities about pregnancy. "Sometimes you get into a thing where every problem looks enormous. When people are very confused I suggest that they write out their doubts and concerns, then figure out which are small and which large. It helps to sort out the big from the small. Then ask each other which can be worked through. When you can verbalize your problem, your partner may be able to offer a different perspective that lets you resolve your doubt."

Gajer often observes a pattern which other psychologists also have noted: partners may have an unspoken agreement to remain undecided. When one decides in favor of pregnancy, the other comes up with a reason against it. A few hours or days later, they both change their minds and switch sides. If you think switching is the pattern in your own case, it helps to review the feelings you had before you changed sides. If you and your partner can discuss why you have an unconscious agreement to switch back and forth, you may be able to work out a solution.

As a basic approach to help decision making, Gajer advises that both partners ask themselves these questions and then discuss their responses together.

Why might you want a child?

What do you think pregnancy will be like?

How do you *imagine* yourself with a child?

What do you expect from your partner?

How would you like to see the responsibility shared?

Are these reasonable expectations?

Are your expectations fairly well matched?

How do you each feel having a baby will affect your relationship?

If you already have children, what will a new child mean to them?

Psychologists also suggest that discussing ideas about child rearing can help couples make a decision. Talking over what you want for your children and your attitude toward their upbringing can bring out both fears and desires. At the very least, it helps to negotiate these issues before the child is born so that when the time comes parents can avoid being caught in a power struggle to determine how the child is brought up.

Another way to help resolve ambivalence is to get some feeling for what it's like to raise children; observe and talk to mothers, fathers, and children you know. Offer to take care of friends' children. Volunteer at a local nursery school.

A final issue to consider is: imagine your future *without* a child, and describe how you envision your life.

Single women involved in an ongoing relationship must face the same issues when thinking about pregnancy. However, those who are not involved in a steady relationship and are contemplating having a child on their own will have some additional problems to solve. Think about these questions.

What support system is available in your community?

How would you support and care for a child?

Where would you live? Who, if anyone, would you live with?

How do you think having a child will affect your future relationships?

As the child grows up, what do you expect will be important to you in the future in terms of your career and other interests?

All of these questions can help you get at your underlying feelings about parenthood. The point of writing out a list of pros and cons isn't to tote up the winning side, but to discover what you really feel about the situation. Dr. Jeppson comments, "Even when the cons outnumber the pros, you may still have a gut feeling that you should do it anyway. And it's this gut feeling that you're trying to get at. List making may clear up some of the confusion and let you recognize your deeply felt desires."

If, after working through these questions, you are still in a quandary and filled with anxiety, Dr. Jeppson suggests using relaxation techniques to calm yourself and reach your deeper emotions. It's difficult to come up with a good decision when you are worried and overanxious. Any form of meditation or physical relaxation can help. When your autonomic nervous system is calm you can trust that the unconscious part of your brain will continue working on the problem. When you are relaxed it will present you with a solution.

"Have faith that you really know what's best for yourself and know a good solution," says Dr. Jeppson. "Making a decision is a creative act, and like any creative act it benefits from your imagination as well as the rational part of your mind."

If you are honest with yourself, you may discover deeper feelings about pregnancy and children than you knew you had. Like one woman who recently had lost her mother, you may find that you want to have a baby because you want to *be* a baby. "When I really got to my emotions I realized that I wanted my boyfriend to take care of me—and if I had a baby he'd have to take care of us both. I didn't especially like this feeling and decided that this was not a good reason to have a baby."

If you don't make a conscious decision but stop using contraceptives—you may have decided to have a baby. If you feel you can't decide but continue to use contraceptives—you have chosen not to have a baby, at least for the time being.

If you do decide to have a child, Dr. Jeppson advises, go with your decision wholeheartedly. Every emotion needs an action to reinforce it. What you *do* feeds into the way you feel. So make plans, read books about childbirth and child rearing, research childbirth classes, work out your finances and career adjustments. When you take action after making a decision, you feel less confused and less ambivalent.

CHOOSING THE RIGHT TIME

Most couples do eventually choose to have children. Although there has been a decline in the number of children per family, the proportion of couples who have children has increased since the turn of the century.

As important as the baby decision is, the decision about *when* to have a baby is almost as crucial. Are youthful vitality and energy the most valuable characteristics for new parents, or are maturity and stability? Most people say that money and work most influence timing of children. But even more important than these issues, in terms of creating a successful family life, is personal development.

Maturity

The road to maturity seems to be a circle—from the blurred dependency of youth in our original families, we have to learn to be independent and selfish, to put ourselves and our own needs before the wishes of our families, to break away, to live for ourselves. "The happiest day of my life," said a thirty-five-year-old woman long enmeshed in her original family, "was when a friend accused me of being selfish. I knew that after ten years of therapy I had finally accomplished something."

Only when we successfully complete this emotional breaking away, according to family therapists, do we have a good chance of uniting in marriage and raising our own families. At that point, we are ready in a positive sense to once again put the needs of the family before our own personal needs.

What we've learned from family therapists is that the best time for pregnancy is when it's right for you. And what we've gained by the trend toward older parenthood is not an answer, but an option.

Age

Despite the trend toward delayed parenthood, most people still marry in their early to mid twenties and have a baby within the first three years of married life. And it is this same group—married couples between their second and fourth anniversaries, often with a new baby—that is most vulnerable to divorce. Current statistics say that about 40 percent of all marriages end in divorce—and the numbers peak among young married people who have one or two children.

Theories about how adults mature psychologically offer a partial explanation. Various investigators of the adult life cycle define the ages between twenty-two and twenty-eight as a period when young people try to fit themselves into the established adult world. Men and women both try to imitate and satisfy their parents in what Gail Sheehy calls the "I should" phase of life. Marriage and parenthood may help you *look* like an adult, but often they are like playing house. When reality sinks in, things can get tough.

Husbands and wives often begin to drift apart as they evolve into their own adult identity. As age thirty approaches they become more conscious of themselves as individuals and search for ways to fulfill youthful promise.

These natural personal changes are harder to manage when you have young children, because a child's needs must be met before your own. It's difficult to serve yourself and also satisfy those who depend on you. As one psychiatrist summarized, "Children do not make good parents."

By age thirty, however, most of us have managed to separate fully from our original families. We know more about ourselves and what we want out of life. We are more ready to settle down and create lasting relationships—in short, the thirties seem an ideal time to marry or start a family. Statistically, the older you are when you marry, the better the chances that the marriage will last.

The longer you remain married before having children, the greater the odds that you'll stay married. Waiting until your thirties or forties to have a baby gives your marriage time to gel. Older parents tend to have more patience and sympathy, and certainly they have more experience in life. They are likely to have a stronger sense of their own identity and worth, so that their own growing pains are not tied up with their children's.

Here is the trouble spot: this is also a time when careers become important. If the decade between twenty and thirty is the time for making mistakes, the following decade is the time to get things done. The thirty year old has some life experience, a sense of identity, and a sense of purpose. Is there time and energy left over to have children? Can babies be added to all the demands of the energetic thirties?

Younger or Older?
There are undeniable benefits to postponing pregnancy. Perhaps the best part of starting a new family late in life is the fullness it brings to the parenting experience. At any age, mothering an infant is hard round-the-clock work. But one mother who had her first two children in her early twenties and her last one sixteen years later at the age of forty, considers age an advantage. "I'm no longer too proud to take a nap when I'm tired, or to ask for help when I'm overwhelmed. I can also afford to pay someone else to clean the house while I spend time just watching the baby and playing with her.

Now it seems to me that the most important thing in the world is the great art of learning to crawl or to blow bubbles."

On reflection some social observers have discovered flaws in this rosy picture. The major problem associated with delayed parenthood is medical—it becomes more difficult to become pregnant when you are past the age of thirty, and many women who have postponed pregnancy find that their fertility is compromised. One problem is that what you choose today may not be what you want in the future. Nancy Goldsmith decided not to have children because of various family circumstances. Her husband had a teenage son by a previous marriage who was feeling rejected by both his parents. Their financial status was precarious. She had come from a broken home herself and dreaded the possibility that her own marriage might break up and she would have the responsibility of rearing a child on her own, making all the mistakes that her own mother had made. All of these were legitimate reasons for Nancy to decide against parenthood. While her husband wanted more children, it was not a pressing need, and he went along with her decision. Ten years later all of these obstacles to parenthood had ironed out. With maturity came stability, and a strong desire to bear children. But she was by this time forty-two years old and unable to conceive.

The best advice from experts is if you plan to delay pregnancy, seek a fertility evaluation. If the evaluation indicates that you have a fertility problem you can receive early treatment, giving yourself a much better chance of later pregnancy. Even if fertility is intact, however, there is always a risk that you might have trouble becoming pregnant as you grow older.

Career planners also point out some difficulties with delayed childbirth. Established careers are often more demanding than entry-level jobs. If you have a child when you are just starting out to work in your twenties, you can probably count on a job with regular hours and no travel. You can gradually build up experience and contacts. Then, in your thirties, when your children are a little older, you can plunge wholeheartedly into work and quickly move ahead.

From an economic viewpoint, older couples generally make more money, but they also spend more money. If one drops out of work to care for an infant it can severely shock the budget. But if you have a baby when you're young and perhaps just beginning a career, it may be easier to build a baby into your budget. Family watchers suggest that for younger parents the money works out without major impact.

Psychologists have brought up some additional problems. It may be harder to change your lifestyle later in life. Having a child represents change, which can upset the balance a couple has achieved. When a husband and wife have enjoyed many child-free years, they may find it more difficult to adjust to the radically diminished time together with a demanding new baby sharing the house.

They also may be faced with staggering college tuition fees at a time in life when they are thinking about retiring, or when there are added financial concerns about their own parents growing older.

All of these pros and cons add up to one thing: the best time to have a baby is when you personally feel that it's right for you. You can, and should, weigh the various components of the decision-making process, and judge them against your instincts. What you decide may not be right for your sister or brother, or the couples who live next door. But it will be right for you.

Combining family responsibilities with work, for both men and women, is the challenge of the 1980s. And certainly the decision about when to have a baby can be a difficult one for couples trying to seamlessly fit together work, marriage, and parenthood. But in some ways, it's an easier decision today than it was even ten years ago.

Today there are fewer "shoulds" about when to have a child. So when a man and woman decide to have a baby—regardless of their ages—it is because they feel the right time has arrived. Each couple chooses according to its own needs and desires and with the conviction that the child will be cherished and wanted.

Regardless of the stability of the marriage, or the time of life in which children arrive, having a baby is a turning point, a shift into family life that represents a genuine crisis. Not only are adults turned into parents, but a family is born, and the family evolves a personality of its own. Every child, from the firstborn on, means a substantial shift in the structure of a family. Every such change should be understood and appreciated before you become pregnant.

CHAPTER 2

HOW A BABY CHANGES
YOUR RELATIONSHIP

AN IMPORTANT PART of the baby decision is projecting what kinds of changes a baby will make in the way you live. If you choose parenthood, what can you expect to happen to your relationship with your partner? As family therapist Sonya Rhodes has written in her book *Surviving Family Life,* "Most couples still retain the illusion that parenthood is joyous and even romantic. The reality, when it finally occurs, is like a cold shower."

According to Rhodes, even when couples consciously choose to have children, and carefully time their arrival, the transformation from twosome to threesome is so little anticipated that even the most eager new parents are caught flat-footed.

Because of the wide variety of family structures on the American scene today it seems prudent to examine—before you become pregnant—some of the profound and unexpected ways a baby might alter your life. Knowing in advance the kinds of stress new families are subject to can help you distinguish serious problems from trivial ones. It can also prevent you from deciding to have a baby for the wrong reasons.

Dr. Rhodes was the first to describe the seven stages that all families, regardless of their size or structure, go through. Each stage requires an adjustment, and every time a family makes a transition from one to another there is heavy stress. Stage 1 is falling in love and establishing intimacy. Childbirth signals the beginning of stage 2 of this cycle, the time when a brand-new family begins. Whether you have a baby at age twenty or forty—after one year of marriage or ten—you can expect to experience this transition. The major change: shifting from a relationship that caters to two adults to a relationship that nurtures a child.

Among the classic social documents of the 1950s is a study that exploded a myth of the American dream family. A group of young urban and suburban couples who recently had become parents were interviewed. In that decade of relative social tranquility, 83 percent of these stable "ideal" couples said they went through an extensive or severe crisis when they had their first child.

Today, no less than in the 1950s, parenthood is still a life crisis in which positions are shifted, values changed, and new roles assumed. How different this stage is from early marriage, when a man and woman first begin to share their lives, and each still retains a certain amount of independence. Having a baby alters forever the nature of this hard-won relationship. Suddenly married life revolves around a third party: the most demanding, helpless human being alive.

Parents begin to make sacrifices in terms of time, money, and attention. They give up some of the pleasures that enriched their marriage—time alone together and energy devoted solely to each other's desires and needs. Life is abruptly changed.

The transition period is eased considerably when couples build a sense of family in the months before and during pregnancy. Before pregnancy, thinking about making changes in lifestyle, expressing your hopes and fears, planning what kind of family life you want; and, later, studying nutrition, reading books about pregnancy and childbirth, taking childbirth classes together, and planning the baby's wardrobe—all are activities that help anticipate change.

Family therapists say that when a baby arrives, new families have to turn inward to nurture the young child. For at this time, the family comes first, and all other obligations are second. But there are problems inherent in this careful nurturing of an infant.

Babies alter the delicate balance between intimacy and distance that every couple strives to maintain in its personal relationship. Some psychologists say that all basic anxieties stem from either a fear of being suffocated or a fear of being abandoned by one's own parents. As we grow older, these fears balance out, but most people continue to lean a little in one direction or the other. We choose our partners based on the way their personalities mesh with our basic insecurities, and the parameters of the relationship are ultimately determined by these unspoken rules of how much closeness and how much distance each person can tolerate. A baby throws this balance out of whack.

If one partner needs plenty of room in marriage, having a baby can increase the sense of being trapped. Conversely, if you are afraid of being abandoned, and need constant reassurance from your partner, a baby can be threatening when it seems that your partner's affection and attention are focused away from you and toward the baby.

Family therapists often remind new parents coming for marital counseling that they need to remember to nurture each other, not only the baby. When they say the family temporarily comes first, they mean the whole family—including parents.

Rocky Marriages

When the marital relationship is strong, couples generally come through the stress of adding a baby to the family with flying colors. But when the marital relationship is troubled, having a baby adds immeasurable strain. The bitter experiences of generations of parents and children prove that having a baby doesn't solve marital problems. Yet many couples in dull or quarrel-ridden marriages continue to have children in order to try to salvage threatened marriages.

Babies are used for all sorts of marital machinations. A young wife hopes a baby will bring her husband closer to her and stimulate his interest in home life. Or she's lonely and dissatisfied and sees the baby as self-fulfillment. A husband may believe a baby will make his wife fully committed to him and their home and so unable to pursue a career, go to school, or meet other people. Or he thinks he will have more freedom if his wife has someone else to occupy her affections.

The trouble with these solutions is the baby adds even more stress to a preexisting marital problem. Instead of solving the problem, the child tends to become entwined in its parents' difficulties. The time to work out problems in your intimate relationship with your partner is *before* you become pregnant.

emerge. The psychological impact also disappeared if the child had reached the beginnings of independence at the age of five or six when a younger sibling was born. The wider spacing seems better for parents. If four or more years have passed since the birth of the last child, parents are more likely to treat a new infant with the same special care and attention lavished on the firstborn.

For the overall benefit of the family, according to Kidwell, a spacing of about five years is optimal. It frees the parent from having to meet the demands and pressures of two small children close together in age, allowing parents and children more time together, one to one, in a supportive and relaxed atmosphere.

Even though researchers stress that this information on spacing of births is still inconclusive, considering how many children you want —and how far apart you want them to be in age—should be an important part of your pre-pregnancy planning.

Becoming a parent inevitably creates change and stress, but these changes require accommodations that often prove beneficial. One older woman looking back on her struggles to rear her child alone said, "It was very hard, but I'm certain of one thing: being a parent made me a better person." Many couples have said that parenthood brought them a deepened sense of permanent connection to their partner. The intense bond is not just between parent and child, but between man and woman.

Today trying to define the modern American family in terms of its structure is a losing battle. The growing acknowledgment that women may need more than motherhood and men more than career to feel whole and fulfilled has had a profound effect on the patterns and shapes of families today. These changes are most apparent in the growing number of career alternatives available in the workplace, options that attempt to recognize and accommodate the complex needs of today's parents.

CHAPTER 3

BABIES AND CAREERS

BABIES AND CAREERS are not a natural combination—they don't go together like apple pie and ice cream. Yet in 1983 working wives contributed about a third to three quarters of their families' incomes —proof that, for most families, the wife's paycheck is a necessity, not a luxury.

When a baby first enters the picture, working parents can expect to be overloaded. The basic problem they face is that there isn't enough time for everything—time for children, time for work, time to be alone together, time for themselves as individuals. Over the long view, working parents do have certain advantages. But in the early years of parenting they need to adjust careers so that for the time being the family can come first.

These adjustments—in terms of career planning and finances— often have to be negotiated and planned far in advance. If you wait until pregnancy, or worse, if you wait until the baby is born, pressure may force you into decisions that are not to your best advantage.

Adjustments might include cutting back hours, negotiating for a leave of absence, foregoing promotions that involve extensive travel, or even changing jobs.

In the past decade working mothers expected to pursue their careers and bring up their babies at the same time. A career woman I know used to get up at dawn to work around the house and spend time with her three-year-old daughter before dropping the child off at nursery school and heading in for work by 9 A.M. She raced home at 5 P.M. to cook dinner for her husband and child, supervised household help, made sure she attended every function at her child's school, and gathered her little family together on Friday evenings for a trek to their weekend cottage. Three times a week she religiously jogged around the local exercise track before going to bed. Her husband worked nine to five and occasionally baby-sat on Saturday mornings while his wife was shopping.

Finally, just before she was ready to be dragged off to the funny farm, the legend of Supermom exploded like a falling star.

Today although more than 60 percent of all mothers work, and almost half of these working mothers have children under the age of six, many women have come to realize that they can't do everything themselves. Working couples with young children are like pioneers in an uncharted landscape. Settling the conflict between work and family life, and equitably distributing the work load, is a difficult and experimental task. It often involves changes between husband and wife, and also between each partner and his or her employer.

Part of the difficulty is that the social support systems—employers, psychologists, and families—are slow to recognize the reality that most families find themselves in, namely, the need and desire of both parents to work outside the home. Despite new evidence, most male specialists in child development still hold that the needs of a young child are best met through its mother. Their views contrast sharply with female child-development experts who point out that this bias for mothers is unsupported by current studies in child-development literature.

There is no hard evidence that young children suffer when their mothers work, and no evidence that routine separations from the mother blunt a child's development. The research does strongly indicate that stable, caring relationships with adults—a mother, father, or another responsible adult—are vital for children, and that an optimal environment can be achieved in numerous ways. The crucial variable is not who, but *what kind* of care is provided for children.

Pat Libbey, co-director of the Career and Family Institute, a nonprofit Minneapolis organization that advises corporations on the needs of working parents, has said, "It all comes down to what these parents should do; when they should have children, whose career should take precedence and when; and how to give home and children the time and devotion they need." Magazines and newspapers and television programs across the nation have experts digging for answers, but in the last analysis each family struggles to provide its own answers. We are slowly coming around to the idea that every couple will have to work out a combination of family and jobs that works best for them.

COPING WITH GUILT

Working mothers have to be brilliant jugglers, keeping all the balls in the air at once. Yet even those who have found original ways to cope wonder if the strenuous demands on their energy are costly to their children, to their careers, and to their marriages. Says Judith Langer, a New York City market researcher who observed discussion groups of first-time moms, many of whom had or wanted careers, "They mention the word 'guilt' almost as often as the word 'baby.' "

Langer, writing in *American Demographics,* found that while many women today have the freedom to choose, the price seems to be self-doubt. "Many wonder, 'Am I cheating my employer? Am I cheating my family? Am I cheating myself?' "

The working women Langer talked with felt guilty about leaving their children and also guilty when they didn't miss them. Those who chose to stay home felt guilty about not working. Other anxieties included guilt about baby-sitters, about not giving enough to their husbands, about husbands helping out too much, about taking time for self, about not working hard enough or working too hard at the job. "The result," says Langer, "is that many mothers feel highly vulnerable to charges that they have somehow fallen short in their efforts."

Couples with the advantages of two hefty paychecks and excellent job opportunities feel particularly guilty if they both continue working after they have a baby, because they know they might be able to get along on one income for a while.

Men, too, have uncertainties about career adjustments and family life, and even advertisers have begun to play upon their guilt feelings. One computer manufacturer recently introduced a TV campaign showing that fathers would have more time to spend with their kids if they installed an automation system at the office. Some family men look for jobs with regular hours and little travel to ensure time at home when their children are young. Yet the reality of the workplace seldom matches their desires.

A man who insists on these adjustments at work may sacrifice promotions and raises. Yet change must start somewhere, and it usually starts with the individual person willing to put himself or herself on the line. Before there are broad, sweeping changes in the way employers view employees who are also fathers and mothers, some parents will have to make demands and take risks.

One young attorney took such a gamble, announcing to his seniors that he would be unavailable for the nighttime sessions and Saturday hours which were common in his office. "I expected the roof to fall in," he said, "and it did. They argued and threatened and basically said that it would be impossible. I stuck to my guns, to the extent that if we couldn't make an adjustment, I would look for another job. They finally agreed to try it for a while. That was two years ago, and I've still got my job. But there have been problems. Some of the other attorneys in the office resent me. And I'm not the guy who will make partner anytime soon. But as far as I'm concerned, it's been worth it."

ARE WORKING MOTHERS "STRESSED OUT"?

When researchers first began to study stress in men they theorized that high-powered, demanding jobs might be linked to such illnesses as heart disease. However, some recent studies show that housewives, especially those with young children at home, are significantly more anxious and depressed than working husbands. When the two were compared, there was little question that housewives suffer more stress. The studies indicate that a mother who works, especially if she has a high-powered job, may actually suffer less stress than her at-home counterpart. When she does become "stressed out," the source of the stress is likely to be at home, not on the job.

"So what else is new?" asked my next-door neighbor, confined at home, tending to two toddlers and two other children in school. "Every mother always knew that little kids drive you nuts. Now they proved it."

What they actually proved is even more interesting than the well-known fact that "little kids drive you nuts." The new research suggests that work and children do go together, and that work itself can be nurturing to mothers.

According to various sociologists reporting from Wellesley, Columbia University, and Princeton, a woman's psychological well-being is enhanced by her involvement in an interesting occupation. A national study conducted by Alma Baron, professor of management at the University of Wisconsin, found that the need for personal fulfillment, as well as money, fuels a woman's willingness to take on the dual task of home and job.

Apparently when the personal fulfillment angle is missing, and a woman works strictly for the money, the positive effect of the job is diminished. Those working mothers who suffer the most stress, according to Dr. Leonard Pearlin, sociologist at the Department of Human Development and Aging at the University of California-San Francisco, are the ones who don't see life getting better. These are mothers doing dreary jobs that don't interest them, forced away from their children often with unsatisfactory day care, working because they must or staying home because it's expected of them.

The key to whether a working mother becomes overstressed seems to be whether or not she enjoys her work. Interesting work seems to act as a shield against pressures at home. Researchers also noticed that the more roles a woman plays, the better her mental state may be. According to the Princeton group, women who have up to five roles function better than women with fewer roles; more than five seems to produce an overload. A woman with five roles might be someone who is married and has children, works at a part-time job, studies for an advanced degree, and sings with a choral group.

There is some conflicting evidence when it comes to women who fulfill three particular roles—wife, mother, and provider—and no others. Those three roles in combination seem to put extra pressure on women to be Supermoms. It may be significant that all three functions primarily involve satisfying others—husbands, children, employers—rather than satisfying the emotional and psychological needs of the woman herself.

Symptoms of stress appear to intensify when a woman is unable to make satisfactory arrangements for child care. If she is career-oriented, it may be very rough for four or five years until the child goes to school. But we know that people withstand stress more easily when they see it as temporary, and knowing that it will come to an end relieves much depression.

OPTIONS IN STYLE

One interesting aspect of the two-career effort is the marital and family issues that surface as couples try to work out their household arrangements. Who stays home when the baby-sitter is late or when the kids are sick? Who goes to school conferences, buys birthday presents, and takes the kids to the dentist? No matter what kind of child care arrangements you can afford, you cannot pay someone to be a psychological parent. Parenting is a passionate career—a career that demands a major investment of time, energy, and commitment for at least the first five years of a child's life.

In some ways parents who both work outside the home are in a good position to plan together. They both have outside responsibilities and home responsibilities. They both would like to sleep through the night and both are tired at the end of the week. They are in similar situations with similar needs, and therefore in an ideal position to negotiate with each other to share the demands of parenthood.

In this sense family life serves to bring independent husbands and wives closer together. Because so much time is spent away from home, family time is cherished and there's less tendency to take the family for granted.

Unfortunately it doesn't always work out so smoothly. A 1982 study conducted by Thomas Juster, director of the Institute for Social Research at the University of Michigan in Ann Arbor, showed that husbands average fourteen hours' worth of helping out each week—three hours more than was the case a decade ago—but wives are still stuck with most of the housework and child care duties. As one economist said, "These couples may have three careers, but the women are doing two of them."

Surprisingly, the majority of women are remaining quiet about this inequity. Only 42 percent of those surveyed said they wanted their husbands to help more. Sociologists believe that some working women hang on to the housework to preserve their feminine identity. Certainly, all of us, finding ourselves in the midst of change, cling to old habits learned early and familiar behavior patterns that have been passed on for generations, even when it comes to house-work.

The hardest part of establishing new role patterns is that there is no special formula. Young working couples contemplating preg-nancy may have to depart from traditional family styles to search for their own patterns. The most refreshing part of their search is that they can examine different solutions and keep the ones that work.

Reduced Work Schedules
Instead of one partner giving up work altogether, some parents try to scale back the number of hours they work. An enormous desire for part-time work emerged in all of the sessions conducted by Judith Langer. A few women in her interview sessions had managed to arrange shorter days or shorter work weeks without changing jobs. Others were willing to switch to a lower corporate level to have shorter hours. Split-shift parenting was another approach: some women took evening jobs while their husbands cared for the children at night. At-home businesses were established in an at-tempt to merge child care with the workplace. And some shopped for the rare work situation which would accommodate two or more mothers who wished to try a job-sharing arrangement.

Unfortunately many jobs simply won't permit this kind of flexi-bility. And even if they do, you may have to pay a professional and financial price. The loss of income and promotions may be worth it, however. And many times a woman has quit her job because of overload, and later, after she is missed, found that her former em-ployer is willing to negotiate a part-time schedule for her.

Women with reduced work hours often find that they get just as much accomplished as working full-time. Some admit, however, that the arrangement causes problems for other employees and sometimes clients and customers.

Reduced working hours need not always require lower family in-come. When their first child was born in 1975, for example, an ar-chitect married to a psychiatrist bought a large house and each set up practice on a separate floor and worked at home. They found it easier to share such duties as shopping and housecleaning and child care. They saved the expense of renting office space, and today their

combined incomes are twice what they used to make and they have
had the pleasure of seeing their children grow up.

The trend for professionals to marry each other—lawyers marry
lawyers, dentists marry dentists, and psychologists marry other psychologists—also offers some unusual opportunities for parents to go
into business together.

One Parent Stays Home

In the midst of all this shifting and sliding in work schedules, another trend has emerged: for a particular period of family life,
women—and some men—are taking time off from their careers to
raise families.

Whether it's Mom or Dad may depend on a number of factors:
whose career will be hurt more by temporarily dropping out of the
work force; which parent's job can provide the family with more
financial security; and even more important, who is actually willing
to take on the job of full-time homemaker.

This new breed of parents does not see parenthood as a cultural
role; nor do they see themselves locked into full-time parenting for
a lifetime. They make different choices for different periods of their
lives. Instead of one role, they choose a series of roles, allowing
themselves maximum flexibility. They say, "Now I'm concentrating
on parenting. Three years from now I'll still be a parent, but I may
concentrate on something else."

The danger in "taking time off," according to one father who tried
it, is underestimating how much work, time, and emotional commitment babies require. In his case, he elected to take a year off to stay
home with the new baby and write a novel at the same time.

"What a laugh," he says now, almost eight months later. "I
should have figured if it were possible to take care of a baby and
write a book at the same time, half the new mothers in America
would be best-selling novelists. The person who decides to stay
home with a baby should accept that he's not going to get anything
else done. It's a full-time job."

When this temporary leave-taking from careers first began, it was
usually women who did it. Lately, however, as women have become
more accustomed to being in a corporate atmosphere, it's anybody's
guess who might have the greater talent or desire to deal with the
children on a day-to-day basis. Thanks to the pioneering efforts of

working parents, it is becoming increasingly easy to shift traditional roles.

BEST JOBS

The careers that seem most compatible with raising children are those that allow you maximum control of your work schedule. Who is sitting in the bleachers after school watching their kids play ball? Who goes to open house at nursery school? Who takes a morning walk in the park, strollers and teddy bears in tow? Real estate agents, free-lancers, sales reps, and lawyers in private practice, among others.

Free-lance workers such as commercial artists, consultants, and direct mail marketers have the most control because they can work at home and still attend to child-raising duties. Since some of their work can be done outside of the usual nine-to-five business day, they might be able to work at night or while children are napping.

Writers as a free-lance group will stand up in a nationwide chorus and sing out "not so"—concentration can snap like a frozen twig, they say, making them vulnerable to the slightest distraction, and a house with a baby in it is full of distractions. But, theoretically at least, it could be accomplished if you have the discipline of a Samurai and a mind like a medieval fortress to defend you against interruptions.

For all of its possible advantages, free-lancing at home has other drawbacks. Income is often erratic, and worries about cash flow are common.

Would-be parents who are teachers, travel agents, designers, and retail buyers have some excellent advantages. These are jobs whose skills do not need constant updating. A temporary leave of absence will not leave you stranded miles behind your colleagues, which means that new mothers and fathers can temporarily drop out of work to spend time with their infants without losing professional ground. These jobs also have more flexibility in terms of how you get to the top than most corporate endeavors.

Colien Hefferan, an economist who studies families for the U.S. Department of Agriculture, believes that families are finding unique ways to adjust to conditions of economic change and uncertainty. Speaking to *Scholastic UPDATE* in November of 1984, Ms. Hefferan suggested that current changes evolving in the workplace may help families cope. "More workers than ever are in jobs that deal with information, in such fields as education, research, social work, and marketing items by telephone. Unlike factory and construction jobs, for example, jobs in the growing 'information sector' allow parents some flexibility in their schedules. In the future computers and other advanced information technology may permit many parents to do their jobs at home."

WORST JOBS

In a May 1985 issue devoted to child rearing in modern society, *Money* magazine concluded that the least desirable occupations for new parents include investment banking, on-staff journalism for magazines, newspapers, or television, politics, and restaurant management—all jobs where eighteen-hour days are considered normal. Highly competitive law, accounting, and advertising are fields that demand total commitment to your job when you're starting out. These careers usually work best for couples who have postponed parenthood until they are well-established at work.

Alternatives

If you're in a career that demands wrenching trade-offs between job and child rearing, you might consider a mid-life career switch. Or you might consider changing employers. Seek out an employer in your field whose business approach blends better with the demands of career and parenthood. Ask at interviews about company policy on such issues as parenting leaves and subsidized day care. Only about five hundred major corporations operate day care centers for employees' children. Many more either help pay for or aid parents in locating independent child care facilities. A few of the big five hundred: Hewlett-Packard, IBM, Merck, Procter & Gamble, 3M, and Stride Rite.

Self-Employed

Another tactic is to go into business on your own. In certain professions the high-pressure demands of major firms can be exchanged for the more flexible atmosphere of a one- or two-person independent practice where you can set your own pace.

WORKING WHILE PREGNANT

Before you become pregnant it's a good idea to consider how pregnancy itself will affect your ability to do your job. In general, if you are healthy and your job does not involve heavy lifting, you can plan to work for as long as you feel able.

Researchers have found no evidence to prove that working women are at greater risk than nonworking women for childbirth complications. However, every pregnancy is unique. Two healthy women working at identical jobs may have different capacities.

When you stop working is something that you must decide with your obstetrician. The following is an approximate guide: if your pregnancy is uncomplicated you can probably work until the end of your eighth month. If you hope to work until labor begins, you should be examined and evaluated by your doctor weekly during the last six weeks.

If your job is physically or emotionally demanding, you should probably stop six to twelve weeks before your due date. If you are expecting twins, you should also stop working at least twelve weeks in advance.

Rather than quit work on a specified date prior to your due date, it's better to leave your "stop work" date open and continue to work as long as you can. That way, if you or your doctor miscalculated your due date, or if the baby is late, you won't use up weeks of precious maternity leave before the baby is born.

Most women are physically able to return to work four to six weeks after a vaginal delivery, and six to eight weeks after a cesarean section, provided there are no complications.

These guidelines do not apply to women who have a history of complications associated with pregnancy and childbirth. Nor to those pregnant women who have a preexisting disease such as diabetes, or those who are carrying multiple pregnancies. (See Chapter 14.) Depending on the extent of the problem, it's possible that you may be able to continue working for several months. In some cases, however, you may have to abandon work completely while you are pregnant.

BENEFITS AT WORK

If you become pregnant, how will your pregnancy affect your job status? By law, pregnant women are protected against discrimination on the job. The only factor your employer can consider is your ability to do your job. Legally you cannot be fired or forced to resign, nor can you be forced to go on leave as long as you can still work. If you are in line for a promotion you cannot be refused it because you are pregnant.

You are also entitled to the same disability benefits as every other employee at your workplace. For example, if your employer reassigns other partially disabled employees to lighter work, he or she is obliged to do the same for you. If other employees get their jobs back after they have recovered from a disability, you are also entitled to return to your job after childbirth.

These are your rights under the Pregnancy Discrimination Act, passed in 1978 as an amendment to Title VII of the 1964 Civil Rights Act. They apply to every business that employs more than fifteen people.

Unfortunately, although this law specifically prohibits discrimination because of pregnancy, childbirth, or related conditions, prejudice against pregnant women still exists in the workplace. Such prejudicial treatment may be overt or subtle. A pregnant woman might be passed over for promotion because her employer feels her baby will interfere with her total commitment to the job. On a more direct level, she might not receive specific disability benefits granted other employees temporarily disabled by accident or illness. While the first example is difficult to prove, the second can usually be rectified.

Before you can claim your rights, you need to know exactly what kind of disability protection your employer offers to all employees. Disability benefits vary from company to company—ranging all the way from lavish weekly payments to no benefits at all. If your company does not provide disability benefits, you may qualify for full or partial temporary disability benefits from your state. However, not every state provides such coverage, and payments vary significantly.

Disability payments cover the period of time from when you stop working to have your baby until you return to the job following delivery. In addition, any health insurance plan for employees must pay pregnancy expenses on the same basis that it pays other medical expenses. If you do not return to work, however, you usually lose all benefits.

If you believe that pregnant women are unfairly treated where you work, you have several courses of action open to you. Some discriminatory practices are the result of ignorance of the law, and speaking to your personnel director or union representative may bring your company's policies into compliance. Your chance of success is improved if you join together with other women at work and express your concerns as a group.

If your company does not comply, you still have recourse to government agencies. To determine your rights and the legality of your claim, contact your state's human rights commissioner, a local chapter of NOW, the American Civil Liberties Union, or the federal Equal Employment Opportunity Commission.

LEAVE FOR CHILD CARE

The Pregnancy Disability Act requires only that pregnancy-related disabilities be treated like other short-term disabilities. In other words, while you have the same rights as other workers in your company, you are not legally entitled to any special benefits that might help your needs as a new parent. A few states—California, Montana, Connecticut, and Massachusetts—have laws requiring special benefits for pregnant employees, but the Justice Department recently has urged the Supreme Court to strike down these state laws, saying that the law forbids discrimination either against or in favor of pregnant employees.

Unlike more than a hundred other countries, including Canada, France, and West Germany, the United States does not guarantee job-protected time off to new mothers. A diverse group of lobbyists, including the Children's Defense Fund, Association of Junior Leagues, the American Civil Liberties Union, the United Auto Workers, and other feminist, labor, and children's groups, have joined together to try to change that. Studies by Dr. Sheila B. Kamerman and Dr. Alfred J. Kahn, co-directors of Columbia University's Cross National Studies Program, show that only 40 percent of new mothers have access to any maternal benefits, and those who do rarely receive full wage replacement and more than six weeks' leave.

The experts vary on their proposals for an optional parenting leave. Dr. T. Berry Brazelton, a nationally known Boston pediatrician, suggested a minimum of four months to allow parent and child to complete the bonding process. Dr. Edward F. Zigler, director of the Yale Bush Center Advisory Committee on Infant Care Leave, prefers six months to allow the family to adjust to the stress of a new baby.

What sorts of leaves are employers granting? Brief and mostly unpaid, according to a national survey of 420 major industrial, financial, and service companies conducted by Catalyst, a New York organization dedicated to increasing the productivity of men and women in the workplace by resolving family problems.

Of the companies surveyed 51.7 percent offered unpaid maternity leave; only 7.4 percent offered paid leaves. Unpaid paternity leaves were offered by 36.8 percent of the companies, although men rarely took advantage of them.

According to the study, 45 percent of mothers are back at work within two months; women in managerial jobs go back even sooner. Such women often reported back to work from home, with daily phone calls, mail drops, and reports delivered to the office—usually without pay.

Most women surveyed said that they would prefer three months' leave. They also said they would like policies that allowed them to work four days a week for a given short interval, then make a gradual transition back to full-time work.

Hope for the Future
There is some hope for improvement in the future. Employers are becoming aware of the changing face of the American work force—with women expected to make up 56 percent of the work force by 1990. After putting so much effort into recruiting women, companies will have to find policies that will help keep them. New arrangements in terms of leaves and benefits are being examined.

The Yale Bush Center Advisory Committee on Infant Care Leave, composed of some of the country's most eminent authorities on child care, has initiated a new study to investigate the possibility of a national policy that would guarantee leaves of absence for new parents.

As a result, Representative Patricia Schroeder, Democrat of Colorado, has recently introduced a bill to establish a national parental leave system. The measure would mandate eighteen weeks of job-protected leave for employees who have a newborn, newly adopted, or seriously ill child. It would also require six months' leave for workers with short-term disabilities arising from pregnancy.

Whether or not the bill passes, the coming together of such a prestigious group as the Yale-Bush Committee, along with other blue-ribbon panels, indicates that these family issues are finally being recognized as serious and growing problems in our society.

If your decision to become pregnant includes juggling two careers and one baby in the same family, the time to start your balancing act is now—before pregnancy. Such a commitment requires flexibility, negotiation, and a willingness to compromise. The questions to ask yourself: What are your employer's views on parenting? Are you happy in your present job, or is it time for a change—before you become pregnant? What pregnancy benefits are you entitled to from your job? Should one of you plan to take some time off after the baby is born? If so, who, and for how long?

The problems faced by working parents are greatly eased if they have access to reliable, affordable child care. Right now, quality child care is so difficult to find that it is an issue that all who are contemplating starting a family today must concern themselves with in advance of pregnancy.

CHAPTER 4

PLANNING FOR
CHILD CARE

IF YOU PLAN TO GO BACK to work after giving birth to your child, the time to start looking for satisfactory child care is before you become pregnant. So scarce is the availability of quality child care many day care centers report that they must turn away parents with three-year-olds who have been on the waiting list since before their children were born. At the Child Development Center, a model child care center in San Francisco, the director reports a waiting list of more than two hundred children for thirty-six spaces. This is not an unusual situation. Similar reports filter in from centers around the nation.

The dramatic increase in the number of households in which both parents work makes quality child care the issue of the decade. Nearly 60 percent of all mothers are working, and 20 percent of these mothers are their families' sole providers. While parents work, who takes care of America's children?

Right now, the answer is day care centers, relatives, housekeepers, the lady next door. And the facts yield one overriding conclusion: child care, as described in a recent editorial in the New York *Times,* "is a hodgepodge of services and stratagems inadequate to a galloping need."

Different families have different needs, and to some extent child care will always remain a "hodgepodge" of different components. But each component can be improved on. Presently there are no federal guidelines on minimum standards for child care. On a state level, some states have minimal standards for day care and others have no licensing requirements at all. A proposed Child Care Opportunities for Families Act, supported by a broad spectrum of organizations, is trying to create some standards in the field by building on the potential of many services already in use. Proposals are under way to upgrade child care standards across the board and also to experiment with different forms of child care. These include experimental full-day kindergartens in local school districts, and community child care in partnership with local businesses.

The most profound and widespread problems facing child care in general are staffing and regulations. The low salaries of care givers are bringing unqualified people into the field. To combat the problem, professionals in the child care field have set up a voluntary accreditation system for early childhood programs and offer a training course that gives people credentials in child development.

Cutbacks in public assistance have made good, affordable group care even more scarce than usual. Infant care is especially hard to find. The average family can afford to spend about 10 percent of its gross income on child care, but in fact it's often much more costly. Services for infants may cost as much as $175 a week, beyond the budgets of most families. In New York City, a two-career couple can easily spend $8,000 to $12,000 annually for quality child care.

Planning in advance how you will provide round-the-clock nurturing for your baby while you are working can save you enormous difficulty later on. At first, you may believe that you should sacrifice everything to afford an in-home caretaker for your child, but in fact this may not be your best option. To make a good decision you need to examine all the options available in your community, and this takes time.

Whatever type of child care you select, if both parents work full- or part-time you are eligible for the child care tax credit. This is true even if one parent is actually looking for work or is a full-time student, and the other parent is employed. Unfortunately this credit is greatly limited in dollar amount and does not provide much financial relief for working parents.

TYPES OF CHILD CARE AVAILABLE

Private Care in Your Home
In many ways, finding someone to take care of your child in your own house may be the best arrangement, especially in the first two

years. A child feels secure in a familiar, consistent environment and will receive personal and consistent attention. From a parent's point of view, this option is clearly the most convenient—no transporting the child, toys, or paraphernalia is necessary, especially if time is short due to a hectic schedule. If a child is ill, someone will be there and neither parent has to skip work. And if you are unexpectedly held up by job or traffic, or have to work odd or longer hours, you have a definite advantage with home care. The major disadvantage, of course, is the high cost. Home care options include nurse-housekeepers, baby-sitters, au pairs, and nannies.

If you can afford it, a nurse-housekeeper can be hired. In addition to salary, transportation costs are normally included, as well as certain meals. Child care, basic housekeeping, and often some cooking are expected. The biggest problem most parents report is inconsistency. Helpers often have children of their own, which means that numerous events can cause them to be late for work or unable to come in.

Live-in help is also a possibility, and sometimes cheaper since you are also providing room and board. A forty- to forty-four-hour work week is the usual agreement, which includes private room, bath, and use of telephone. If the arrangement calls for five days' living in instead of seven, the family gets some privacy on weekends; but this option tends to cost more since the helper needs to make weekend living arrangements.

Baby-sitters who do no housework can be hired on a regular basis, although full-time sitters who tend to earn less than housekeepers are rare.

The au pair system is an import from Europe which is becoming popular over here. Au pairs are usually young women who enter the United States on a visitor (not worker) visa and are treated as part of the family during their year or two stay. In exchange for child care and light housekeeping, they receive airfare, full room and board, at least fifty dollars per week, and usually weekends off.

Child care is less of a problem when grandparents and other family members are nearby and available to help. But in the United States today it is estimated that only one in five families have this luxury. When relatives help care for your children you usually save money. But even if your relative goes so far as to decline a regular salary, you should provide carfare, meals, and other extras or gifts.

If you are paying a relative for child care, even one who lives with you, you are still entitled to the child care tax credit (unless you claim the relative as a dependent in your household).

Parents with two high incomes can consider hiring a nanny who may live in or out. The term "nanny" implies professional experience or credentials in the child development area—a degree in child psychology or education, for instance, or experience as a pediatric nurse. Nannies are full-fledged professionals who are hired strictly "on the books" and receive all appropriate benefits. There is at least one private nanny school which supplies highly trained baby nurses at equally high prices. Even if you can afford it these individuals are scarce.

Household help is sought in a variety of ways. Friends and colleagues may have suggestions. Employment agencies that specialize in household workers may be the best source. Even when an employment agency tells you that it checks references, you must double-check yourself. Always make up a list of questions you want to ask, and speak personally with the applicant's previous employers.

Group Care Options
Basically there are two types of "outside the home" child care facilities currently available: day care centers, which provide care for a fairly large group of children, and family day homes, in which a few youngsters are cared for by a woman in her own house.

Day Care Centers
Day care centers, which by definition accommodate seven or more children, come in all sizes and styles. They're found in churches, schools, meeting halls, office buildings, and storefronts and are normally open from 8 A.M. to 6 P.M. They may be run by individuals, community groups, churches, schools, and other public agencies, parent groups, or employers. There are also such nationally franchised chains as KinderCare and Child World. Some programs are similar to family day homes—games, storytelling, playtime, naps, and meals. Others resemble nursery schools, group children by age, and emphasize educational activities.

The best type of day care offers organized and creative activities, equipment, educational toys, nutritious meals and snacks, and on-call medical staff. Unfortunately this sort of quality care is expensive and much too rare to satisfy the ever-growing need.

Many centers will not take infants and only 15 percent of day care kids are infants or toddlers. Private centers often charge $140–$240 monthly. According to a Department of Health and Human Services study, $280 is average at centers for babies under age two. However, costs can be much higher, especially in big cities.

In some areas there are publicly subsidized centers which are aided by federal, state, and local sources. These can be free or cost up to forty-five dollars a week, depending on need. Generally, however, the number of slots available are so inadequate to the demand that only a fraction of those families who qualify are able to take advantage of these facilities.

Aside from the price, parents wonder how sending their children to day care facilities will affect their development and happiness. Many childhood development specialists believe that good substitute care more than adequately supplies the needs of infancy and toddlerhood. Small children seem to benefit from interaction with one another, learning more quickly and developing early skills in communicating and getting along with others. In fact, one new study by Alison Clarke-Stewart, professor of social ecology at the University of California at Irvine, showed that children going to organized day care centers and nursery schools were six to nine months more advanced than children given home care in their own or another's home.

A concurrent study by Kathleen McCartney of Harvard University showed that children's sociability, language skills, and intelligence were most developed in day care centers with experienced directors, a high ratio of staff members to children, and ample opportunities for staff members to interact individually with each child.

The children whose development was most advanced had the advantage of high-quality day care and also came from stable families that gave them love, support, and stimulation. Conversely, day care seems to have a negative impact when the family is under financial and other stresses.

The operative words in the positive findings are "quality day care." While mothers and fathers shopping for day care centers worry about the much publicized incidents of child sexual abuse, it's more common for children in low-quality day care to suffer from not enough time spent reading and playing with the child.

The yellow pages of your local telephone book provide a full listing of day care centers under "Day Nurseries & Child Care." Many cities have a child care office, operating out of the mayor's office, which will provide lists of local centers. Check in your telephone directory under the listing of your city's government offices.

The Junior Leagues of America also operates a referral service. Check to see if the league has a local chapter in your community.

Family Day Homes

More than two thirds of group day care kids are in family day homes; the Children's Defense Fund estimates there are over five million such slots. Family day homes usually take in two to six children and tend to have more flexible hours than do centers. They are often run by a neighborhood mother who can pay close attention to the children. For this reason, the homes are especially popular for babies and toddlers, especially since many day care centers will not take infants.

At their best, this type of environment is the closest thing to home and family, with the additional advantage that your child has the opportunity to interact with other children. In contrast to day care centers, with larger groups of children, family day homes offer an opportunity for personalized, consistent care from a single care giver, perhaps throughout a child's preschool years. However, the quality of care in some homes may be low, especially if the person in charge is overworked, and if there are no organized activities.

The cost of family day care is widely variable. With overhead costs low, these homes can cost as little as $100–$280 per month. But with child care needs escalating, a study by the Department of Health and Human Services recently estimated that the figures were closer to $400–$600 monthly.

Corporate Care

Only eighteen hundred of the nation's six million employers offer child care services to their workers, but that is a threefold increase in two years. The government has tried to encourage corporate involvement in child care by establishing tax incentives for employers who aid their employees in the search for adequate child care arrangements. Under the 1981 Economic Recovery Tax Act, child care expense money offered by an employer as part of an established child care benefits plan does not have to be declared as taxable income by the employee. As far as the employer is concerned, anything spent for child care assistance under this arrangement is treated as a legitimate business expense.

While corporations are traditionally slow in getting started, the Employee Benefit Research Institute suggests that child care may become the key employee benefit of the 1990s.

The nonprofit, nonpartisan group that surveyed the labor force reported in its May 1985 edition of "Issue Brief" that "among the relatively few employers who maintain child-care programs, the advantages include a decrease in the rate of employee turnover and absenteeism, heightened morale and motivation in the work place, and the increased ability to attract employees."

As desirable as these programs are, the report noted a surprising trend—when employers did offer such programs, only 4 to 10 percent of employees used the program at any given time. One reason for the low use rates is that employers, fearing liability suits for substandard care, lean toward facilities with licensed providers—while parents seem to dislike institutional care.

The research institute suggested that employers consider alternatives, such as financial aid for in-home care or family home care. Another option would be donations to neighborhood child care centers. Some companies, in lieu of their own day care center, pay for part or all of their workers' day care costs. Some contract with child care vendors for a certain number of spaces for employees. Others provide information and referral services. Occasionally two or more companies have combined their resources to open a center. Only an estimated four hundred U.S. firms have opened their own on-site facilities so far, mostly hospitals and universities and a few high-technology firms who compete for highly skilled workers.

Still, only 1 percent of businesses presently offer any sort of child care help. But the situation is likely to change. A new generation is moving into corporate management, and they know firsthand about conflicts of work and family. Given the changing nature of family and work in our society, couples today looking ahead to having children can hope for an improvement in the picture.

Community Services

Churches are currently the largest provider of early childhood programs, and civic groups are also helping. Many groups, from labor unions to service clubs, sponsor children for a day care scholarship, provide volunteers, or furnish space, materials, and other help. State and local governments can also play key roles in promoting child care. California, for example, has established a network of sixty-one agencies throughout the state to help educate parents regarding child care and to provide technical assistance to care givers. Under a new law in San Francisco, developers of downtown skyscrapers must provide space or money for child care centers. And more plans are being introduced for safely taking care of the children of working parents. New York City provides approximately five hundred day care openings for children of teen mothers who then are able to go back to school. Some communities have begun early-morning and late-afternoon programs in their public schools.

Many parents are taking the problem into their own hands. Small cooperative day care groups are becoming popular across the country. Parents in Reston, Virginia, formed a cooperative nonprofit day care center that now serves three hundred children. A California mother persuaded her employer to sponsor a child care center in a nearby vacant school building. Similar programs are getting under way in various communities around the country as parents join forces to solve their child care problems.

CHECK IT OUT: CHOOSING A CHILD CARE PROGRAM

When you shop for child care of any kind, talk at length with the person who will provide care; look for warmth, understanding, and experience. Ask about her or his philosophy of child rearing. Look over the play area, kitchen, bathroom, and napping space.

The critical factor is the general mood: Do the children seem happy and busy? If there is more than one care giver, are other staff members friendly, relaxed, attentive? What is the ratio of staff to children? Ask about the experience and training of the staff members. Check out the variety of activities offered and look for a good mix of indoor and outdoor programs. The people are your primary concern, and the setting is secondary, but look for pleasant surroundings and good basic equipment.

You might want to ask if a particular facility is licensed; but keep in mind that only about 10 percent of existing child care facilities are, and this should probably not be your deciding factor.

No matter what kind of child care you are looking at, always talk to other parents who have children in the home or center you are considering. After you have made a decision and placed your child, follow up and occasionally drop in for a visit without warning. Always ask your child how things are going and what he or she did at day care, and listen carefully to what your child tells you.

The real key to finding the right child care for your particular situation is to start looking early, and to cover the field. As you can see, quality situations are rare and waiting lists long. Your ultimate decision should be based on the degree of quality available at a price you can afford. The specific *category* of facility is irrelevant. Even if a family day home is your initial preference, for example, you may find an excellent day care facility that surpasses any private home. Or even if you can find a baby-sitter to come in for a specific number of hours each day, you may discover a much better situation in an "out of home" facility where your child will benefit from playing with other children and learning interesting preschool skills and games.

A good place to start is by calling the Child Care Information Service 1 800 424–2460. This hotline, sponsored by the National Association for the Education of Young Children, answers questions on all aspects of child care, including types of care available, costs and state licensing regulations, and referrals to local child care resource and referral services.

Child care, particularly infant care, is at a crisis level in America. Because of the scarcity and need it is appropriate to start considering the issue before you become pregnant, since you may even decide that a major move is your best solution if it brings you closer to a grandparent or relative, or to some other optimum child care situation.

Many prospective parents register their babies for day care before childbirth. But, as we have seen, even that may be too late. Whether you can sign your child up for day care *before* pregnancy is a point as yet undetermined. But you can try. At the very least by doing your research in advance, and making your plans, as soon as you become pregnant you will have already made your choice and can sign your forthcoming infant up immediately.

Once the choice has been made, the next most serious question is how to pay for it. The weekly cash outlay for child care is only one way your budget will be affected when you decide to bring a baby into your life. If you're not already sitting down, grab a chair for the next chapter—money.

CHAPTER 5

THE BIGGEST HEADACHE: MONEY

BRINGING UP BABY is more expensive now than at any time in memory. Years of steady inflation—the high cost of living—is responsible for much of the rise. But there is another. Before the fifties, there was no such thing as a children's "market." Adults made all the decisions and children were not consulted about the clothes they wore (usually scaled-down grown-up garments), the books they read, or what they listened to or watched. Today's kids make decisions, even about costly expenditures. And the expectations of children, as well as of their parents, include such necessities as summer camp, cars for teenagers, and a college education—all luxuries in our parents' day.

Adding 5 percent a year for rising prices, the U.S. Department of Agriculture (USDA) figures that the average child born in 1984 would cost $140,927 to raise to eighteen. Private economic consultants, who use a different economic model than the government does, almost double that figure, bringing in an estimate of $278,399.

If you send your new baby to college in the year 2003 (eighteen years from now), you can tack on up to $116,000. If you're laughing, now is the time to sober up. An important part of the baby decision is figuring out a financial plan. Advance planning should include some analysis, health insurance, savings and investments, as well as disability and life insurance.

Fortunately the above prices don't mean that you actually have to spend that much, although these numbers do supposedly represent average costs. What you spend depends partly on where you live, and partly on what you consider necessities for your child. The USDA says that expenses tend to be higher in most small-town and rural areas, largely because of transportation costs, which make up a whopping portion of the overall child-rearing bill. On the other hand, if you live in a big city, you may opt for a private school, which can add on as much as six thousand dollars a year. A more reliable standard is the relationship between costs per child and family income. According to statisticians the cost of raising a child from birth to age eighteen is approximately four times one year's income. For each additional child the cost is only two times one year's income. In other words, costs diminish rapidly after the first child.

When looking at this ratio it helps to remember that the one year's income we're talking about is the year your child is born. The way things are presently going on the economic scene, you can look forward to increased income through your thirties and forties. If your income is forty thousand dollars the year your child is born, you can expect its upbringing to cost you a hundred and sixty thousand dollars spread out over eighteen years.

Raising kids is still a highly individualized pursuit. You may spend less than is forecast, and of course you might spend more. An important factor: the increase in expenditures does not come all at once. These overall figures are best used to spot the big-ticket stages in a child's life, and preparing yourself to cope with them.

WHERE DOES THE MONEY GO?

How are these hundred-thousand-plus dollars distributed in the bottomless well called child rearing? According to the USDA, it goes like this (assuming an additional 5 percent annual inflation, and also remembering that you can easily double these prices):

Food:	$34,122
Clothing:	10,695
Education:	2,642
Medical care:	7,827
Personal care & recreation:	17,176
Transportation:	22,522

The item that seems clearly out of line is transportation. But when you consider that a child needs transportation to virtually every activity that he or she attends outside the house for eighteen years, it is more understandable.

If we know what the money goes for, the next question is *when* does it go? Which years in a child's life are the most expensive?

Costs for child rearing fluctuate over the child's growing years. Expenditures start high during pregnancy and childbirth, then drop after birth and during the first five years (depending on your baby's child care needs). Food, the largest expense in the child's life, costs little at infancy if you are breast-feeding. Kids actually get cheaper over the next five to six years, if one of you is staying home. But you might have lost income and should also count a financial loss if your career stalls out.

Expenses start to inch up when your child goes off to school. Food and clothing are major expenses for a rapidly growing youngster. Summer camp and weekly lessons in ballet, computers, piano, gymnastics, tennis, and other sophisticated pursuits are almost routine for today's child.

The cash outlay continues to escalate through the teenage years, when kids need spending money, a car, either their own or yours (insurance can more than double), and tickets to sporting events and rock concerts. After seventeen, things really heat up, and the next four years of college is the most expensive time of a child's life.

What you're looking for are ways to reduce the enormous start-up costs—pregnancy and childbirth, and that end-of-childhood whopper—college tuition. In the first instance, a good health care plan, in place before you become pregnant, will offset some of the major costs. Family and friends can help you further, reducing your outlay for such expensive items as clothing and furniture.

And, in the second, the time to start saving for your child's college education is now—as soon as you decide that you're going to have a baby.

BIG-TICKET BABIES

Many financial planners recommend that a couple have at least three months' living expenses put aside in an emergency fund; when you decide to have a child, ideally, you should try to double that amount. This money should be readily available: money market accounts, short-term certificates of deposit, or treasury bills. If accumulating an emergency cash fund is impossible, apply for a five- to ten-thousand-dollar line of credit from your bank. You'll pay interest on the money only if you use it.

With emergency funds in place, prospective parents should start to look ahead for ways to defray some of their start-up costs. Babies come into the world at considerable expense. Costs to get you through nine months of pregnancy, childbirth, and six weeks of postnatal parenting can range from three thousand to more than nine thousand dollars. What you spend depends largely on your health insurance coverage, the generosity of your family and friends in outfitting your baby, the kind and amount of baby furniture, clothes, and toys you purchase, and how expensive your own tastes are in pregnancy clothing.

Medical costs begin with your first prenatal visit to the doctor to confirm the pregnancy. At this time the doctor's fee is usually discussed. Obstetrical bills are usually paid in monthly installments *before* the birth. An obstetrician's fee, which covers office visits and the actual delivery, plus a postpartum checkup, range from $700 to $1,550 and up for a normal delivery, more for a cesarean delivery. Hospital costs are billed separately, as are any special prenatal tests and lab work, such as amniocentesis and ultrasound scans. The sum total of physician and hospital expenses average $2,300 to $4,450.

Roughly two thirds of these costs should be picked up by your medical insurance. If you're even thinking of starting a family, check your health policy *first.* Once you are pregnant it is impossible to switch to a plan with better benefits.

It's unlikely that any policy will cover all of your costs. Charges for the nursery, or circumcising and conducting routine tests for the infant, may not be included in your policy unless you belong to a health maintenance organization where all costs are covered in a comprehensive fee. You may also have to budget additional money to cover routine monthly visits to the pediatrician through the baby's first year.

If you are under thirty-five years of age and have no serious health problems you may trim costs if you choose to have your baby in an out-of-hospital birthing center. Full maternity care costs around fifteen hundred dollars at these centers, and includes prenatal office visits, prepared childbirth classes, a twenty-four-hour stay after delivery, and a postpartum checkup. Most medical insurance programs now cover these alternative birthing centers.

There are many other pregnancy expenses unrelated to actual childbirth. A baby literally comes naked into the world, minus even the most basic clothing needs. And even an infant will need wheels to get around town. Clothing, crib, stroller and car seat, high chair and playpen, formula and diapers all cost money. If you're lucky, generous grandparents, relatives, and friends will get you started with much of what you need. An important thing to remember is to buy ahead gradually while you're pregnant, anticipating that your infant will grow rapidly and be ready for larger sizes almost every month.

Once you are over the financial hurdle of childbirth, and your family has been enlivened by the living presence of your baby, the expenses may ease off temporarily. Unless both of you are working. If so, the next major expense you will encounter is child care.

If you are lucky enough *not* to need paid child care help over the next few years, child-related expenses decline. Continuing to save during this time—money market funds, certificates of deposit and other investments—can help you in the more costly teenage years. After your child starts school your expenses will go up gradually over the next few years, until he or she enters high school, where there is an almost steady outlay of cash. The next major expense, however, is still coming up.

STARTING A COLLEGE FUND

College costs have already increased far beyond most families' ability to pay. In the past three years alone, tuitions have risen an average of 15 percent, while student aid—from private low-interest loans, outright grants, or government-subsidized loans—is increasingly hard to find.

Eighteen years from now, assuming a 6 percent annual increase that financial planners predict in education bills, your child's four-year private college degree will cost an average of $116,000. Sending your child to a public university will cost $40,700.

If it sounds impossible, financial planners say that many new parents will be able to manage these prices if they start a college savings fund as part of their pre-pregnancy financial plan. If you set aside $2,348 a year, with an after-tax yield of 8 percent a year, in eighteen years you will have enough to meet private college bills. If you set aside $822 a year over eighteen years, you'll be able to meet the expenses of a public university.

If these figures make you gulp, financial planners emphasize that the important thing is to begin some sort of systematic savings plan —no matter how modest. Even a few hundred dollars a year turns into a few thousand dollars in eighteen years, a nest egg that can help your child considerably when he or she is ready for college.

There are many ways to achieve an 8 percent return after taxes. You can invest in a tax-free bond fund; the greatest risk in such an investment is that its market value might drop because of a rise in prevailing interest rates. One way to get around this problem is to buy a zero-coupon municipal bond; you pay a fraction of what you will receive when it matures, and the bond pays a fixed return. Bonds are simple to purchase and your investment can range from a few hundred dollars to many thousands of dollars.

If you are in a high tax bracket financial planners also suggest putting some of your income in the child's name and investing it. The income from the investments will be taxed at the child's presumably lower rate—usually nothing at all. There are several ways to make these investments, and it's a good idea to consult a lawyer or financial adviser to make sure that you're making the best choice for your income bracket and not violating any IRS regulations. In general, there are three strategies.

The easiest is an outright gift. Under the Uniform Gift to Minors Account (UGMA) each parent can give a child up to ten thousand dollars a year without having to pay federal gift tax on it. Money cannot be used for what the government terms parental obligations —food, clothing, and housing—but, depending on what state laws allow, it can go toward education and almost anything else you can think of. A gift is irrevocable, and when your children legally become adults, usually at age eighteen, they will be able to spend it as they wish. All that's needed to set up a UGMA is a Social Security number for your child (obtained by applying to your local Social Security Administration office).

A slightly different option is a Clifford trust, with your child named as beneficiary. Any income earned on the money you put into the trust belongs to your child and is taxed at the child's rate. Ten years and a day after the last deposit the trust reverts to you. A third option, a Crown loan, allows you to lend money to your child without charging interest. The loan can then be invested, in your child's name, and interest is taxed at his or her lower rate. You can lend your child any amount, but once you transfer the money to the child's name the money can be used only for his or her needs.

Changes are afoot in these kinds of trusts, and a child's Clifford trust income may soon be taxed at the parents' rate. Check with your lawyer first.

In terms of investments, most parents choose the safe and steady variety. Both time and money tend to be in short supply when children are young, and parents look for simple, easy to manage investments with guaranteed returns: government-backed bonds, treasury bills, or bank certificates of deposit are attractive.

When you're thinking about financial planning over a period of eighteen years, with the goal of a college education for your child, plus a safety net and retirement for yourself, the best thing you can do is seek the advice of a financial planner. You don't have to be rich to benefit from this advice, and many working parents with two regular jobs who feel they are just making ends meet have been surprised to learn that they are worth much more than they think.

INSURANCE NEEDS

A baby brings extra responsibilities for both parents, and two important considerations for prospective parents to think about are disability insurance and life insurance.

Most people have the disability insurance provided by Social Security, but the current top benefit (at this time thirteen hundred dollars a month) probably isn't enough to meet the needs of your family if you are unexpectedly unable to work because of an accident or illness. The company you work for may provide disability coverage, but check to make sure. A pregnant woman is entitled to the same disability coverage as is any other employee in her company, but benefits vary widely from company to company. Check your company's policy to see if you are protected in case you can't return to work when you planned because of childbirth complications. Financial planners say that you should aim for disability benefits that would replace about 60 percent of your pretax salary. If your disability coverage is not up to par, you should think about buying your own policy. Disability insurance is expensive, but you can reduce premiums if you lengthen the waiting period for benefits to start. For example, you may pay a high premium for a policy that begins to pay benefits one month after you are disabled. But if the policy begins three months after you are disabled, the price of the monthly premium may be cut in half.

Life Insurance
It's a good idea for both parents to take out life insurance policies, so that in the event of one partner dying, the other will have enough money to bring up the child. The best recommendation made by financial planners is renewable-term life insurance, which is simple and cheap. Term insurance, however, does not build any equity and each year you start over again.

A family's insurance needs are usually highest when all its members—parents and children—are young. During this early period, term insurance provides five to eight times more protection for every premium dollar than does whole life. And low premiums can usually fit into any budget.

The premiums on term policies increase as you grow older, while the premiums on whole life policies remain the same. An experienced insurance agent may suggest to you some ways to combine high protection when you're young with guaranteed insurance when you're old, and at a price within your budget. For example, one new type of policy lets you move freely between term and whole life as your needs change, without having to cancel old policies or take out new ones.

You can also buy a combination whole life policy with a term rider attached that provides for additional death benefits if you die before a certain age.

Whole life insurance is basically a savings plan, and many experts consider it insignificant because of the comparative low interest rates paid by insurance companies. Consumer advisers on insurance generally suggest that young parents choose term insurance over whole life, and invest the difference. But how you save money is a matter of personal style. If you don't want the responsibility of choosing among investments, or if you find it difficult to put money away without the incentive of a premium that must be paid, whole life may be a good option.

Nor do financial planners generally recommend insuring a child's life as a way to save for college. Again, life insurance is usually not as profitable as other investment strategies.

WILLS

If you are like many Americans, you haven't made a will because you're pretty certain you don't have anything of value. If you have a baby you will have something very precious to leave—your child. If one of you dies, the other automatically has custody of your child. But if you and the child's other parent both die without making a will, the state chooses a guardian for your child. (The state will also decide how to dispose of your property.)

To have any say over your child's future it's vital that you each make a will naming your choice of guardian. When you select a guardian make sure you talk it over with the person you choose. If you don't there is always a possibility that the person you name will refuse the job, leaving it to the court to seek out a substitute.

If you wish you can appoint two separate guardians—one to care for your child, and the other to manage the child's finances. A guardian who handles the money could be a lawyer or banker or a friend with financial savvy. That person has discretion over how the money is spent but must get the court's permission to spend large amounts of money. He or she must also submit an annual accounting to the court. If you want to exercise more control over your child's finances, you can set up a testamentary trust which spells out how the guardian should invest and spend the money.

To make even a simple will you need to hire a lawyer to make sure each of your wills is drawn up properly. The fee will be about $150 each.

When you are attending to all of these matters, financial planners make this reminder: on your various policies add your child's name as a contingent beneficiary.

Because of the astonishing changes in the worldwide economy, raising a family today is more costly than at any time in history. Creating a sound financial plan that can be projected across your child's growing years is an important part of pre-pregnancy planning. If the financial picture leaves you a little weak in the knees, talk to some new parents you know, parents like Ken and Liza: "We spend money like we're printing it in the basement," Liza says. "I never dreamed that I'd pay seven dollars for a pound of cherries just because Jason likes the color. And at the end of every month we're mutually horrified at our cash flow. But the truth is, we don't care. Having Jason is the happiest part of our lives and I don't know how we ever lived without him."

Making a decision about if and when to have a baby, anticipating the changes creating a family will have in your life, making career adjustments and planning for the future are the stepping-stones to emotionally and psychologically preparing yourself for pregnancy. This preparation, once easily assimilated, is more complicated today given the complexities of modern society and the array of personal options open to each of us. In the long run, it's a gratifying process. Having the freedom to choose based on our individual needs, as well as our responsibilities to others, holds the promise of rewarding family life where the needs and potential of each person in the family are fulfilled. Even though the family is no longer a structured social unit with rigidly defined roles, it's an adaptable organism, with a constant purpose: to nurture and protect, to encourage and support growth, to express love.

Hand in hand with practical and psychological preparation for pregnancy goes physical preparation. We know more about health care and fitness today than ever before. We are also subject to more distressing elements from pollution, drugs, alcohol, and smoking. New research coming forth daily has shown conclusively that all of these elements can radically affect pregnancy and the future well-being of our children. It is imperative that a woman contemplating pregnancy consider a detoxifying health program to prepare her body for a healthy pregnancy. The next six chapters are devoted to analyzing your health and fitness and creating a strong, healthy body before you become pregnant.

PART TWO

HEALTH
AND
FITNESS
FOR
PREGNANCY

CHAPTER 6

THE BIOLOGICAL FACTS

HAVING A BABY IS LIKE building a house—you have to prepare a good, strong foundation before you start the actual construction. The foundation from which a baby grows is a woman's egg, or ovum, and a man's sperm. To give a baby the best start in life both partners have to be as healthy as possible before they try to conceive.

To help understand why ordinary properties—alcohol, cigarettes, contraceptives, and other common elements—can have such a devastating effect on the reproductive organs, even before pregnancy, here's a picture of the delicate, human reproductive system and what happens when you conceive.

Conception occurs when two cells, an ovum and a sperm, unite within one fallopian tube in a woman's body. The ovum, no bigger than a grain of salt, is the largest cell in the female body. The sperm is one of the male body's smallest cells. The journey of these two minuscule cells to the place in the body where fertilization usually takes place is through an intricate maze, fraught with obstacles.

MALE REPRODUCTIVE ORGANS

A man's reproductive organs are designed to manufacture, store, and deliver one special product. The product is sperm, and the packaging is a nutritive, protective liquid called seminal fluid.

Sperm are manufactured in the testicles, two small organs wrapped in membranes and suspended in the protective pouch of the scrotum. This vulnerable position outside the body cavity helps keep these important organs cooler than the rest of the body. Theoretically, this somewhat cooler temperature helps maintain a steady production of sperm.

Within the testicles are thousands of tightly coiled microscopic tubules lined with primordial germ cells. When a boy reaches puberty these cells begin to generate millions of sperm every day. Each mature sperm cell has an oval head, a midpiece, and a long whiplike tail. The head contains precisely half the usual number of chromosomes, topped by a cap which houses chemicals to help the sperm penetrate an ovum.

The testicles eject up to four hundred million sperm cells with each ejaculation. Hundreds of thousands of sperm are squandered lavishly in the hope that one will seek out and fertilize the single egg produced each month by a woman's ovaries.

FEMALE REPRODUCTIVE ORGANS

The vagina is the outside passageway to a female's internal reproductive organs. A small, tight valve called the cervix connects the vagina to the uterus. The uterus itself, a small, pear-shaped organ, is suspended within the pelvic cavity by long bands of ligaments. A fallopian tube opens off each upper corner of the uterus. The ends of the two tubes swing free. Attached to either side of the uterus by short muscular stalks are the small, white ovaries, each no more than 1¼ inch across.

Each of the two ovaries houses roughly two hundred thousand eggs that will last until a woman enters menopause. Each month a single ovum matures inside an ovary and works its way toward the surface. About halfway into the menstrual cycle the ovum breaks through the surface of the ovary and the egg pops out, leaving its shell or follicle behind.

The egg falls through space. This is a critical point, for now a slender fallopian tube leading to the uterus must receive the egg in its open end. To broaden the catching surface of the narrow tube, the fringed open end, called a fimbria, splays open like a flower and draws the egg inside. The lining of the tube is like velvet. Millions of tall cells with soft hairlike tips called cilia brush the egg along in undulating waves toward the uterus. The ovum approaches the high reaches of the tube, the one point in the body where it usually can be fertilized.

When a man ejaculates, millions of sperm are ejected from the pocket of the testicles up through a series of ducts. Seminal fluid pouring into the ducts from the prostate gland and adjacent storage areas flush the sperm through the urethra and out the tip of the penis. The sperm must be deposited in the woman's vaginal vault, pass through the tiny opening of the cervix, swim through the uterus, and then reach the fallopian tubes.

It is not an easy journey. The path that sperm must travel is an obstacle course designed to eliminate all but the best. Most of the sperm die instantly, destroyed by harsh acid fluids that cleanse the vagina. Only a few hundred, swimming furiously, make it to the cervix, and even fewer reach the fallopian tubes. Most of the time the sperm are turned back by a wall of mucus that blocks the cervix and prevents bacteria from invading the abdominal cavity. Obviously were this protection sustained all month long, procreation would come to a complete halt. Nature, fortunately, has designed a loophole. For a few brief hours each month, at the exact moment when an egg drops from an ovary, the thick cervical mucus changes into an abundant, fluid stream that sperm can swim through.

Those sperm that get past the cervix now have about forty-eight hours remaining to reach and fertilize the ovum before they die. If they move too quickly, however, they may overshoot the fertilization point before the egg gets there.

Some sperm harbor in little crypts inside the walls of the cervix. Others are entrapped by gauzy mucosal folds within the fallopian tubes. The fine hairs of cilia streaming toward the uterus also work against them.

The hazards of the journey help ensure that only the most perfect, active sperm reach the vicinity of the egg. Nevertheless, a poor quality sperm and egg do sometimes fuse; most of these fertilized eggs stop developing and are lost spontaneously without a woman being aware of the pregnancy.

Both processes—sperm selection by "ordeal" and early, spontaneous abortion—are beneficial, quality-control measures evolved by our species.

Those sperm that journey as far as the fallopian tubes undergo a final transformation. Every mature sperm has an invisible membrane protecting its head and holding its chemicals in check until the right moment. As the sperm swims toward the fertilization point, the coating slowly wears away until the head is bared.

As the egg slowly tumbles through the fallopian tube, dozens of minute sperm rush to meet it. All of the sperm are fully capable of penetrating the egg, but only one can succeed.

To reach the nucleus of the egg, a sperm must first dig through a sticky coating of jelly. Spraying chemicals from its head, the sperm dissolves a hole in this outer layer, only to find another, tougher membrane underneath. The sperm now concentrates its chemicals in a narrow jet and slits a small opening in the shield. At that moment, the sperm locks onto the egg and injects its blob of DNA into the egg.

The membrane surrounding the egg is instantly transformed into a rigid barrier. No other sperm, despite the strength of its chemicals, can enter. If the barrier fails and more than one sperm penetrates, the egg will die from a lethal excess of DNA. Twins are never formed by two sperm entering one egg. Two eggs may be fertilized by two different sperm (fraternal twins), or a fertilized egg may divide into two separate embryos (identical twins). But only one sperm can enter one egg in which a human develops.

When the sperm touches the egg their membranes fuse like two touching bubbles. The nucleus of the sperm now lies inside the egg —one cell of the mother and one from the father have merged into a hybrid cell. In the next few moments the chromosomes of the egg and sperm will match up to form the full chromosome array of the first cell of the new person.

The Sexual Imprint

The moment that the twenty-three chromosomes of the sperm cell pair up with twenty-three compatible chromosomes of the ovum all the properties of a new human life are determined, including its sex. Whether the fetus will be a boy or a girl is determined by which sperm enters the ovum. Although rare aberrations arise, the ovum itself almost always carries an X sex chromosome. Sperm cells, however, are about equally divided between Xs and Ys. If the sperm that penetrates the sticky surface of an egg also carries an X, the baby will be a girl. If it carries a Y, the baby will be a boy.

The fertilized egg continues to move through the fallopian tube. In three days' time it divides into two cells; each cell divides to make four, and again to make eight. At this point the eight-cell embryo is ready for transfer into the womb, where it will cling to the inside wall of the uterus. For the next forty to sixty days the pregnancy will be supported by progesterone manufactured by the empty egg sac (corpus luteum) that is left behind on the surface of the ovary. After that, the placenta will take over the hormonal work load.

LIKELIHOOD OF ACHIEVING PREGNANCY

Many couples believe that the woman will become pregnant the first month after they stop using contraceptives. In fact, even if you have intercourse on the right day and sperm are present when the egg drops off the ovary, conception doesn't necessarily occur. Even under such ideal circumstances, pregnancy is chancy.

The fallopian tube doesn't always catch the egg as it falls. If the egg doesn't make it into the tube, fertilization cannot take place no matter how many sperm are waiting. Rarely a dropped catch becomes fertilized outside the fallopian tube; this is one type of ectopic pregnancy (see Chapter 16), which always leads to early miscarriage. There are dozens of other possible missteps in the game.

Based on experimental studies, scientists estimate that 15 percent of the time the ovum is incapable of being fertilized; and 25 percent of the time it is fertilized, then silently aborts. In addition, a certain number of ova never make it into the fallopian tube. Overall, a couple has only a 20 percent likelihood of conceiving in any given month. With these odds, it may take up to a year for the woman of an average couple to conceive.

Frequency of Intercourse

Should you increase your sexual activity when you are trying to become pregnant? Technically, having sexual intercourse once in a month's time is enough to achieve pregnancy, if that one time occurs during the twenty-four-hour period when a woman is ovulating. Since ovulation is an unseen biological mechanism of the body, however, it is difficult to know exactly when it occurs. Further, no one is sure exactly how long sperm can live within the female reproductive tract before they die.

Although live sperm may be found in the mucus, uterus, and

fallopian tubes up to ninety-six hours after intercourse, there is evidence that their fertilization power lasts only twenty-four to forty-eight hours. Similarly, the egg has only about twelve to twenty-four hours after ovulation during which it is capable of being fertilized. If there is to be any chance of fertilization, these two short periods must overlap.

Researchers still do not know if it's better for a couple to have sex every day, every other day, or every third day to maximize their fertility potential. Ejaculating too often—or too seldom—may lead to problems. A man with a moderate to low sperm count will be relatively infertile if he ejaculates every day because he depletes his volume of stored sperm. On the other hand, if he abstains for two weeks or longer, the sperm in storage are likely to die. The rule of thumb recommended by most fertility experts is that if your usual sexual activity doesn't lead to pregnancy within a few months, try having sex every day. If this still doesn't work, switch to every other day.

YOUR MOST FERTILE DAYS

A woman's most fertile days are during ovulation. Although we know ovulation occurs approximately midway through the menstrual cycle it has very few outward signs. You cannot know precisely when the egg leaves the ovary and enters the fallopian tube.

Menstrual cycles vary considerably among women but normally fall into a pattern somewhere between every twenty-six and thirty-two days. Once established, the number of days between periods stays roughly the same month after month, although it may be altered by stress or illness.

The menstrual cycle is divided into two hormonal phases, controlled by signals from the brain. The first two weeks, called the estrogen phase, prepares the egg; the second two weeks, called the progesterone phase, releases the egg and prepares the uterus for pregnancy.

The cycle begins with the first day of bleeding. In the first two weeks a group of follicles begins to mature in the ovaries; one follicle grows faster than the rest and works its way to the surface of the ovary. (The word "follicle," often used interchangeably with ovum, actually refers to the shell or sac, filled with fluid and an egg, or ovum, floating inside.)

Also during this two-week phase, the thin lining of the uterus grows thicker as it is stimulated by estrogen produced by the follicles. By day fourteen of the cycle the endometrium may be ten times thicker than it was the week before. At the point when the endometrium reaches its full thickness, the follicle bursts open and the egg pops off the ovary. This is ovulation.

The follicle shell is left behind. This remnant, called a corpus luteum, takes on a crucial new task. Under new hormonal signals from the brain and pituitary gland, it begins to secrete large amounts of progesterone. The cycle now enters its progesterone phase.

As the empty eggshell pumps out progesterone, the thickened endometrium grows spongier. If the egg is fertilized, it will pass from the fallopian tube into the uterus and bury itself in the plush endometrium on about day twenty-two of the cycle.

If the ovum is not fertilized, it is absorbed into the body and disappears, and the corpus luteum ceases to produce progesterone. The abrupt loss of hormone causes the endometrium to break down; the walls of the uterus contract and push out the lining. The menstrual cycle is complete as soon as bleeding begins, and in a few days the complete lining is discharged through the vagina.

(If the ovum is fertilized, it begins to secrete an early-pregnancy hormone called human chorionic gonadotrophin [HCG] which signals the corpus luteum to continue sending progesterone to support the uterus.)

The Hormonal Axis

The growth and release of the ovum, and the growth and shedding of the endometrium, are controlled by hormonal signals from the brain. The brain signals the pituitary gland, the pituitary gland signals the ovaries, and the ovaries send hormonal signals back again to the brain.

In women, the signals switch midway through the cycle. And it is this switch that boosts the egg off the ovary and thus controls ovulation.

The Temperature Chart

Some women, particularly those over thirty, begin to worry about fertility when they don't become pregnant immediately. If you want to ensure that you have sexual intercourse on optimum days, you might keep track of your ovulation.

While you cannot know exactly when you ovulate, there are two indirect signs that predict ovulation. One is a change in cervical mucus, which becomes clear and watery during ovulation. When you notice this abundant mucus during the month, you are ovulating.

The second way is by body temperature. In the days immediately *after* ovulation, your body temperature rises slightly. If you take your temperature every morning, beginning on the last day of your period, it should remain relatively low (about 98° F) until about day fourteen of the cycle; then, in response to the increased presence of progesterone in the bloodstream after ovulation, it shifts upward to about 98.4° F and remains elevated through the remainder of the cycle. The temperature will drop again with your next period. If you become pregnant, the temperature will remain elevated.

The drawback of this system of measurement is that the shift takes place *after* ovulation has occurred. Your most fertile days, therefore, are just before the rise. To use a temperature chart as a timing device for intercourse, you must anticipate the rise. If your menstrual cycles are regular, it is relatively easy to predict when the rise is about to occur. Some women show a noticeable dip in temperature just before the upward shift. This dip, if it occurs, coincides with ovulation.

The key to keeping an accurate chart is to record your temperature first thing in the morning, before getting out of bed. Keep the thermometer and the chart on your nightstand, and try to take your temperature at about the same time each morning.

Taking your temperature every morning is a tedious endeavor, and for most women an unnecessary one. If you want the assurance of a chart, however, it's usually enough to keep track for a couple of months until you know approximately when to expect the upward shift. If your menstrual pattern is regular, you will ovulate at about the same time each month.

Home-Testing Kits

A more convenient and more reliable method of predicting ovulation is provided by new home urine tests which let you detect the presence of LH, the hormone released by the pituitary gland to boost the egg off the ovary. The urine test is performed every day for five days, beginning around day ten of your cycle. If the dip stick changes color, LH is present, suggesting that ovulation is *about to occur.*

Home-testing kits are more accurate than the temperature chart, and also more expensive.

Should your temperature fail to rise (or should the dip stick fail to change color) for two or more cycles it's possible that ovulation is impaired and may be at least part of a fertility problem.

BEFORE YOU STOP CONTRACEPTION

After you decide that you want to have a baby, wait three to six months *before you stop contraception* to give yourself time to assess your health and lifestyle and make appropriate changes. (See Chapter 12.) This is the interval in which you should optimize your nutrition and general fitness, and have a medical checkup.

You may also want to change the form of contraception you use. (See Chapter 9.) For example, if you are on the pill, it's a good idea to substitute a diaphragm or have your partner use a condom for at least three months before you try to become pregnant.

The chapters that follow are based on the premise that you have decided to become pregnant but are going to wait a minimum of three months before you try to conceive.

CHAPTER 7

ENVIRONMENTAL EFFECT ON PREGNANCY

IN THE EARLY DAYS of an embryo's life, before a woman even knows she is pregnant, all the organs in the baby's body have begun to form and are at their most vulnerable. Poor diet, smoking, drinking, workplace environment, or drugs could at this early stage cause some damage to the embryo. Hazards may come from either the mother or the father. By the time a woman's pregnancy is confirmed, her partner's heavy smoking, drinking, or some chemical he may work with, as well as certain diseases and drugs, may already have harmed his sperm.

Our new awareness of these effects shows that parents influence their baby's future even before conception. Before you become pregnant you can begin to avoid those things we now know or suspect can harm your baby. (Bear in mind, however, that despite precautions and preparations some babies are born with unavoidable problems. This possibility cannot be completely ruled out.)

SMOKING

Smoking is the most common environmental cause of problems in an unborn baby's development. Smoking negatively affects the spectrum of reproduction—fertility, conception, development of the fetus in the uterus, labor and delivery, and the development of the baby as he or she matures in childhood.

A woman who smokes heavily often gives birth to a baby who is considerably smaller than a baby born to a nonsmoker. Smoking during pregnancy has also been directly related to an increased rate of premature births and stillbirths. Women who smoke have a 25 percent greater chance of miscarriage than do nonsmokers. The effects of smoking during pregnancy are long lasting. Low birth-weight babies born to women who smoke do not appear to catch up later in life. Studies have shown that even at the age of eleven children of mothers who smoked during pregnancy were, on average, shorter and less intelligent than those whose mothers did not smoke. The differences were small, but distinctly measurable.

Increasing numbers of scientific studies show that the elements contained in cigarette smoke can injure the fetus in several ways, some of which are immediately apparent while others develop more slowly and insidiously. Carbon monoxide reduces the amount of oxygen available for the baby. Nicotine constricts the placental blood vessels, diminishing their life-supporting flow. And cyanide, the third element in cigarette smoke, a toxic agent in itself, strips nutrients from the fetus.

Loss of oxygen and vital nutrients may be responsible for many fetal abnormalities, including brain damage. When a pregnant woman smokes only two cigarettes, the fetal heart beats faster and the fetus demonstrates abnormal breathing-like motions—both signs of fetal distress.

There is no time during gestation that the fetus is safe from its mother's smoking. From its earliest embryonic stages of rapid cellular division, continuing through its uterine life, the fetus is ominously threatened by these repeated and cumulative assaults.

New evidence suggests that the damage may begin even *before* pregnancy. For the first time it has been conclusively shown that women who smoke are less fertile than nonsmokers and it takes them longer to become pregnant when they try to conceive. A new survey of pregnant women found that 90 percent of the nonsmokers succeeded in becoming pregnant within six months, but only 76 percent of the smokers became pregnant in the same interval.

The mechanism by which smoking impairs a woman's reproductive capacity is unknown, but if smoking damages the competence of the reproductive system, perhaps by breaking down circulation to the uterus, that effect could carry over to a future pregnancy even if the woman stops smoking before pregnancy.

Heavy, passive smoking—that is, the smoke a woman breathes in from other smokers—can also reach the fetus. And after being born the baby can continue to suffer from the smoking of those around it. A nursing baby may receive nicotine in breast milk or by inhaling smoke. By breathing in smoke from adults a child is made vulnerable to a host of ailments, including ear, nose, and throat infection, bronchitis, pneumonia, asthmatic attacks, and decreased lung efficiency.

A new survey by the National Institute of Health Sciences has determined that living with people who smoke increases a person's risk of developing cancer. And these are not only the cancers typically associated with smoking, such as lung cancer. A dramatic increase was also noted for such cancers as leukemia, not previously linked to smoking.

The risk goes up according to how many smokers a person lives with. People who lived with one smoker faced a cancer risk 1.4 times higher than those who did not live with a smoker. The risk was 2.3 times higher for those who lived with two smokers. And 2.6 times greater for those who lived with three or more smokers. The researchers reported among people who lived with three or more smokers, the chances of developing leukemia were nearly seven times greater than for people who did not live with smokers.

In light of this information, it is clear that to protect their child *both* parents should try to stop smoking, or at least reduce their intake, several months before pregnancy and permanently stay off cigarettes once pregnancy is achieved. Whenever possible, pregnant women should also avoid staying too long in a smoky atmosphere.

One important reason for stopping well in advance of pregnancy: breaking bad habits can be stressful, and the early stages of pregnancy aren't the best time to be adding stress to your life. Further, stopping for most people takes time; only a few stalwart souls can stop suddenly and quickly. Further, you may be unaware of the exact time you conceive—and even in the early days of pregnancy smoking is dangerous to the fetus.

Try to stop smoking completely. If you cannot give up smoking without help, contact your doctor or join a self-help organization.

ALCOHOL

Alcohol is the second most common environmental hazard to the fetus. A woman who drinks heavily during pregnancy (five to six drinks a day) has a significant risk of giving birth to a baby with fetal alcohol syndrome, a cluster of severe physical and mental defects caused by alcohol damage to the developing fetus. The most common major abnormalities are growth retardation, facial abnormalities, brain damage, abnormal development of various body organs, including heart defects, and poor muscle coordination. Mild mental retardation (I.Q. is usually 60 to 75), hyperactivity, and learning disabilities are also common.

While particular defects vary from baby to baby, children of alcoholic mothers who drink heavily, especially early in pregnancy, are likely to suffer the most severe abnormalities. From 40 to 50 percent of the babies of heavy drinkers are born with fetal alcohol syndrome.

Most of the other affected babies, including many born to moderate consumers of alcohol, may suffer more subtle fetal alcohol effects.

Studies have shown that pregnant women who consume about ten drinks a week, which is classified as moderate drinking, doubled their risk of having a low birth-weight baby. Low birth-weight babies may have difficulty breathing, poor temperature control, low resistance to infection, and a reluctance to feed.

Even a woman who drinks occasionally may place her baby at risk. Doctors at Columbia University recently reported a significantly higher rate of miscarriage among women who consumed as little as two drinks a week.

When you drink, the liver detoxifies the alcohol and converts it into usable energy. The liver performs this conversion process slowly; any excess alcohol overflows into the bloodstream and is eventually carried to every cell in the body, including the placenta, from which it passes to the fetus. Experimental studies have shown that when pregnant monkeys receive a concentrated form of alcohol, the umbilical cord pales and collapses; in most cases a full hour elapses before the cord can recover its normal condition.

Researchers believe this interruption in circulation between mother and fetus may explain mental retardation in babies whose mothers drink heavily during pregnancy. (It's estimated that fetal alcohol syndrome may be the most common cause of mental deficiency in the United States.) Other explanations are also feasible and the answer awaits further, more definitive studies.

Can you drink at all during pregnancy? The U.S. Food and Drug Administration (FDA) has handed down this guideline: more than six hard drinks each day presents a major risk of serious problems to the fetus; two to six drinks per day carries a substantial risk of lesser abnormalities. *There is no known safe level of alcohol consumption below which no risk is present.* The advice of many obstetricians is to give up drinking altogether—before becoming pregnant. Studies with animals have shown that alcohol may damage newly fertilized ova, and that the embryo is endangered after even a single episode of heavy drinking at the time of conception.

If you are unable to stop, reduce your intake to the lowest amount possible. Dangers may be increased if you are at risk from other factors, such as smoking. A good diet, while helpful in every other way, will not make up for the harmful effects of alcohol. There is some evidence that sporadic drinking is especially dangerous; avoid binges completely so that blood alcohol level will at least be low at all times.

Fortunately many women dislike the taste of alcohol when they are pregnant. If you need help to stop drinking, contact your physician or the nearest chapter of Alcoholics Anonymous.

When Men Drink

Heavy drinking appears to affect a man's sperm in several ways. Alcoholic men often have depressed sperm production. If the liver is damaged by alcohol it cannot clear used hormones, which causes small amounts of female hormone to build up. These excess hormones depress both sperm production and potency. Alcohol also causes an inappropriate release of the hormone prolactin, which has deleterious effects on sperm production.

Experiments with mice have also shown that alcohol given to male mice before mating increased the risk of embryos dying in utero. It seems at least possible, therefore, that some miscarriages might be attributable to heavy drinking by the male partner in the weeks or months before conception.

CAFFEINE

No one yet knows for certain whether the caffeine contained in tea, coffee, chocolate, and some soft drinks is harmful during pregnancy.

Studies in animals have shown that high doses of caffeine were linked to numerous abnormalities in newborn rats, mice, and rabbits, but these findings have not been shown to have a correlation in humans. The FDA has issued a warning to pregnant women to modify or stop their consumption of caffeine-containing foods and beverages, but it also states that evidence of harmful effects is inconclusive. Scientists know that caffeine interferes with the body's ability to absorb and use certain nutrients, specifically iron and some forms of protein. Caffeine also crosses the placenta and is distributed to all fetal tissues.

So, although harmful effects have not been proved, directed by current information most authorities advise that a pregnant woman stop consuming caffeine or limit herself to one or two cups of coffee or other caffeine-containing drinks a day. But unfortunately those who are hooked on caffeine usually consume much greater quantities. It's estimated that 13 percent of pregnant women drink five or more cups of coffee each day.

OTHER DRUGS

Marijuana, cocaine, LSD, and similar drugs may affect sperm and inhibit fertility, as well as damage the fetus. Glue sniffing by a pregnant woman may also affect the fetus's development.

Substances in marijuana are known to remain for weeks, and even months, in body tissues, including the testicles. Marijuana may cause an inappropriate release of prolactin, which may affect a man's fertility.

Babies born to drug-addicted mothers are also addicted and suffer withdrawal symptoms at birth. This distressing and difficult-to-treat problem may result in an infant's death. Physicians fear that many women who use cocaine underestimate the danger of this drug, and that their babies, like those of heroin addicts, will suffer developmental problems and long-lasting brain dysfunction.

It's important for a woman who uses any drug regularly to seek her doctor's advice before trying to conceive.

Prescription Drugs

The drugs thalidomide and diethylstilbesterol (DES) have made people aware of the potential danger to the fetus of drugs taken during pregnancy. Even drugs taken near the time of conception can be hazardous, since it is in the first few weeks of life that a baby's vital organs are forming.

Although scientists have identified several drugs that pregnant women should always avoid, they are still not sure what proportion of birth defects are actually caused by these substances. The cause-effect relationship is difficult to trace because women often do not realize they are pregnant during the first few weeks after conception, so they may fail to keep track of the drugs they take at that time. A further complication is that certain defects, such as heart and kidney problems or mental retardation, may not become apparent for months or years after the child is born—and a woman may not remember what drugs, if any, she took during pregnancy.

To settle some of the unanswered questions about the effects of drugs on the unborn, a number of scientific groups are continuously tracking data on birth defects. According to an article by Pauline Post, "Drugs and Pregnancy," published in *FDA Consumer* magazine, this ongoing research has shown that the fetus is most susceptible to drug effects during the first trimester of pregnancy, when cells are rapidly dividing to establish organ systems. Recently it has been shown that a woman who in the first three months of pregnancy takes Accutane, a drug used to treat severe acne, has twenty-five times the normal risk of having a baby with a major malformation.

Many other commonly used drugs also have been associated with birth defects. Such antianxiety agents as Valium, Librium, and Miltown may cause the development of a cleft lip or cleft palate in a fetus. Anticonvulsant drugs are also associated with similar defects. Most women with seizure disorders, however, must continue to take anticonvulsants during pregnancy, despite the risk, because a seizure is more dangerous to the fetus than medication is. Before becoming pregnant a woman with a seizure disorder should consult her physician; she may be able to take a safer form of anticonvulsant.

Some antibiotics and anti-infectives, particularly tetracyclines and metronidazole, should be avoided. Several others, however—including penicillin, ampicillin, and cephalexin—seem to be safe in pregnancy.

Aspirin should also be avoided during pregnancy. Large doses of aspirin taken during the first few weeks of pregnancy might cause such defects as harelip and cleft palate. Aspirin also interferes with blood clotting; large doses taken in the last month of pregnancy may cause bleeding in the mother or in the newborn. If you become ill and need medication to reduce fever, acetaminophen is preferable to aspirin.

During pregnancy no drug can be considered absolutely safe. Risk depends on the type of drug, the amount taken, and the stage of pregnancy. It also depends on your own susceptibility, which is governed by such ambiguous variables as your genetic makeup and environment (diet, smoking, drinking, and pollution).

Before you stop contraception and try to become pregnant, it's a good idea to stop using all nonprescription drugs, including medicated creams and sprays, aspirin, and cough mixtures. If you are taking prescription drugs, consult your physician before stopping.

If you take medication for a chronic condition, such as diabetes or epilepsy, you should also consult your physician before attempting to conceive. A good diet will help counteract some of the adverse effects of many drugs but, before you try to become pregnant, your doctor may decide to alter or adjust your medication, or send you to a specialist.

Have a dental checkup and any necessary dental work done before you become pregnant. After you conceive, if you must visit your dentist or physician for reasons unrelated to pregnancy, mention that you are pregnant, so that you do not inadvertently receive potentially harmful medication. (For further information on dental care, see Chapter 16.)

Men and Drugs

In experimental studies, drugs given to male animals before mating proved to have deleterious effects on offspring. So a prospective human father should be aware of the potentially harmful effects of the drugs he takes while his partner is trying to conceive.

A host of medications taken on a regular basis—including aspirin in large doses—has the potential to temporarily hamper fertility in men.

Certain drugs may affect the quality and/or quantity of a man's sperm. Antihypertensives, antidepressives, and hallucinatory drugs can disrupt the brain's hormonal signals to the sperm-generating center of the testicles. Narcotics such as morphine and opium derivatives are known to release the hormone prolactin, which also blocks hormonal signals.

POLLUTION AND STRESS

Several groups of pollutants have been linked to infertility, miscarriage, and fetal damage. Radiation, chemical substances such as toluene (a solvent found in glue), and certain metals such as lead have all been implicated (also see Chapter 8).

Traces of lead and other pollutants are unavoidably present in the air you breathe and in the food you eat. Even organically grown produce may pick up traces of insecticides, pesticides, or other chemicals from water and soil that has run off from neighboring land. There has been no solid evidence credibly linking these common environmental factors with problems associated with pregnancy and birth, but such multiple interconnections, while difficult to unravel, are considered possible.

A wholesome diet will provide much protection against ordinary pollutants. For example, if you eat a diet adequate in iron, calcium, copper, and zinc, you will absorb less lead than someone whose intake of these minerals is low.

Effects on Sperm Production

Stress, heat, and altitude, to mention only a few factors, can all affect sperm production. As sperm cells grow and mature, they become increasingly sensitive to toxic agents from the environment. Therefore, a man suffering from environmental stress may continue to produce sperm, but the cells may be sluggish or deformed. Sometimes only some of the sperm-producing tubules are affected while others remain relatively free from toxic damage.

Deformed sperm may be the only symptom a man shows. Two separate hormonal systems control sperm production and sex drive in men. If one is damaged, the other may continue to work perfectly. The sperm-generating cells are the most sensitive and most likely to become damaged; while the cells that make testosterone—the male hormone that governs sex drive—can sustain almost any abuse. Therefore, a man may have poor sperm production and still have a perfectly adequate sex drive.

Stress

In general, stress, anxiety, and tension have a deleterious effect on sperm production. Emotional stress alters the functioning of the lower brain (hypothalamus), which in turn affects the output of various hormones. In animal studies overstressed male rats showed diminished fertility, and young mice in crowded cages showed delayed puberty. Even though these effects are well documented, most researchers believe that only severe and prolonged stress, not the ordinary wear and tear of daily life, will affect human fertility. The trouble with this view is that it's difficult to measure the total amount of stress in a person's life. Stress events accumulate in modern life, with subtle and compounded effects.

If you or your partner take drugs to reduce stress, try to cope with it by less potentially hazardous methods. It may help simply to write down the causes of stress or talk things over with your partner, doctor, minister, or a friend. Consider taking a class in yoga or an exercise class at a local Y or health club. Gentle, rhythmic exercise, such as swimming, cycling, or walking, is a good way to release tension.

Heat

Heat is thought to interfere with sperm production. Truck drivers, for example, who sit for long hours literally on a "hot seat," may have a low sperm count. Welders working inside boilers or storage tanks may have surrounding heat of up to 120° F. In these cases sperm production is often severely depressed. Likewise, the man who regularly takes a long soak in a hot tub or sauna may show a depressed sperm count. Tight briefs that hold the testicles close to the body all day can also contribute to overheating. When humidity is excessively high, the body cannot effectively evaporate its heat through perspiration. As a result, the body retains heat, with deleterious effects on sperm production.

However, most experts in male infertility believe that heat exposure would have to be continuous over a long period of time to affect sperm production in any important way.

More serious are new reports that newly pregnant women who take long hot baths or saunas may be endangering the embryo. One study from Temple University reports that the increased temperature from hot baths or hot tubs will damage a baby's nervous system within the first thirty days of conception. Evidence from animal studies suggests that high maternal temperatures result in reduction of blood flow to the fetus. In uncomplicated pregnancies short stretches in a sauna or hot tub are probably not harmful if the temperature is less than 102° F and exposure is limited to ten minutes.

In general, when a woman is trying to become pregnant, it's best for both partners to avoid prolonged exposure to heat.

Altitude

Relocation to a significantly high altitude—say, from sea level to five thousand feet or higher—may result in a temporary reduction in sperm production. When deprived of oxygen, sperm-generating cells seem to go into a resting state. The higher the altitude, the more pronounced the effect. Conversely, divers working below a hundred feet also may have depressed sperm counts, possibly due to the high saturation of oxygen from oxygen tanks.

Environmental hazards may have an insidious effect on our reproductive capacities. Cigarette smoking, drugs, and alcohol—the most dangerous toxins for a developing fetus—have become so pervasive that any couple considering pregnancy must also consider how to detoxify themselves before conception. Fortunately, as dangerous as these substances are, they are elements well within your control. Ridding your system of toxic elements before pregnancy is perhaps the most important thing you can do for the future health of your baby.

There are other hazards, however, that are more difficult to counteract. We are surrounded by an increasingly toxic environment and routinely exposed to chemicals unheard of even twenty years ago. This is particularly true in certain occupations. Some of these risks are discussed in the chapter that follows.

CHAPTER 8

ON-THE-JOB HAZARDS

YOUR JOB MAY BE DANGEROUS to your health, and to the health of your unborn baby. Toxins are all around us, but the most concentrated and dangerous hazards are in the workplace. Over sixty thousand chemical substances are in common commercial use in this country, and we still don't know what long-range effect most of them have on humans.

Humans may absorb toxic substances through the skin, through the digestive system, and through the lungs. The effect may be sudden and severe—blistering of the skin or lungs, vomiting, dizziness —or it may take years to develop. Lung disease, most cancers, and liver diseases develop after latency periods of fifteen to forty years.

Such effects seldom can be traced to one singular toxin. While scientists generally test substances for toxicity one at a time, in real life our bodies usually must contend with more than one toxin at once. Combined, two or more hazards can produce an effect greater than either one alone. The classic example is asbestos. Asbestos workers are at risk for cancer, and asbestos workers who also smoke have the highest risk of all.

When we talk about toxins we are usually talking about the risk for cancer. However, the reproductive systems of both women and men are especially vulnerable to toxins, and reproductive health hazards are among the most important issues in health today. A reproductive hazard is any agent that endangers the male or female reproductive system, or the developing fetus. Infertility in either sex, spontaneous abortion early in pregnancy, or a baby born with birth defects might all be caused by environmental toxins present in the workplace.

HOW HAZARDS AFFECT PREGNANCIES

Environmental hazards can attack directly or indirectly. In men chemicals may directly kill spermatogonia, the sperm-generating cells that line the testicles. Or they may invade the nucleus of the spermatogonia and rearrange DNA. These spermatogonia may die or may produce inferior sperm. Should this damaged sperm succeed in fertilizing an ovum, birth defects could occur. Finally, and most dangerous of all, the spermatogonia may begin to divide into sheets of abnormal cells without definition. This is cancer.

In women toxic substances can cause menstrual disorders, sterility, or loss of sexual drive, either by directly damaging the ovaries or by altering hormonal balance. Toxins may also damage the genetic material in ova, leading to spontaneous abortion or birth defects.

In the fetus, toxins that do not apparently harm an adult can cross the placenta and damage a fertilized egg or fetus. A developing fetus is especially susceptible to environmental hazards because cells are dividing and growing rapidly. Substances that cross the placenta—called teratogens—are particularly dangerous during the first three months of pregnancy, sometimes so early on, that the woman may not be aware that she is pregnant.

Toxins can also disrupt the pattern of growth later in pregnancy. If the toxin is strong enough, the pregnancy may end in a spontaneous abortion. If the fetus survives, the child may have a low birth weight or physical developmental or behavior problems, some of which may not show up until years later.

The list of industrial waste products is so long that it is impossible even to determine the number of chemicals that might affect reproduction. Spurred by the chemical disaster in Bhopal, India, in December of 1984, Congress, and more recently the Environmental Protection Agency, have been working on programs to help states and communities identify potential chemical hazards and develop emergency procedures for coping with leaks.

Unfortunately the strategy consists merely of developing a list of pollutants that could be hazardous in accidental situations. There is an inevitable lag between the discovery of a toxic substance and the translation of that discovery into action. As Kenneth Pelletier has pointed out in his book, *Healthy People in Unhealthy Places*, identifying toxic agents in the workplace is essential and must proceed in a methodical manner, but it is dangerous to delay action in workplaces where there is already clear evidence of hazards.

One peculiar aspect of reproductive hazards is that if they are considered at all they are usually defined as a woman's problem. And in a twisted manner they have been used to discriminate *against* women. For example, women are denied certain hazardous jobs (coincidentally, also high-paying) because they pose a threat to their reproductive systems. In this way, they have been kept out of many high-paying jobs "for their own good." The truth is, any job that threatens a woman's reproductive system also threatens a man's reproductive capacity.

Attorney Lori B. Andrews cites this example in an 1982 article she wrote for *Parents' Magazine:* a federal appellate court scrutinized the protective policy of the Olin Corporation which prevented women from working with lead or other materials suspected of harming a fetus. These jobs were invariably high-paying. Women workers challenged the policy on the grounds of discrimination, offering scientific evidence that showed that a fetus was also susceptible to harm if the father was exposed to lead or other hazardous materials. Their point: Reproductive hazards are often used as excuses to penalize women workers and permit management to avoid cleaning up the workplace. If the company really cared about the safety of workers' offspring they would eliminate the hazard or exclude fertile men as well.

Despite these legal precedents guaranteeing women the right to make their own choices about work, employers continue to claim that since women are childbearers they need special protection. The argument seems hypocritical because a fetus can be adversely affected through the exposure of either its father or mother, meaning that companies that claim they are protecting fetuses by excluding women are indulging in high-level double-talk. Women may be excluded from hazardous high-paying factory jobs, for example, but they're not usually excluded from equally hazardous low-paying traditionally female jobs, such as those in the health industry.

Obviously women's groups do not advocate that women be placed in jobs that endanger either their fertility or the safety of their babies. What they *are* bucking for is accurate information about job hazards for both men and women. And this information is hard to come by.

Working people need credible scientific data to judge the risks that their jobs pose to their ability to become parents of a healthy child.

RISKY JOBS

The most widely publicized risky jobs are those involving radiation. In the 1950s, shoe salesmen who used fluoroscopes to demonstrate correct fit became infertile. Since then the effects of X rays on sperm production have become well known among the general public.

Radiation appears to do its worst damage on the sperm-generating cells that line the testicles. (All the other cells of the testicles usually escape damage, which means that sex drive is unaffected.) Some of these spermatogonia may survive and continue to produce sperm, but the sperm also may suffer from the radiation. Sperm may be incapable of fertilizing an ovum, or they may carry defective chromosomes.

Spermatogonia damaged by radiation seem to have some ability to heal themselves. Five men rendered sterile in a radiation accident at a nuclear plant in Oak Ridge, Tennessee, eventually recovered their fertility after forty-one months. However, even if the spermatogonia revive, their DNA code may be altered.

Doctors, dentists, and X-ray technicians are most obviously at risk for radiation poisoning, but all men and women should be guarded from unnecessary exposure to radiation. Anyone going for X rays should have the reproductive organs shielded with lead plates. People who work with radiation should be monitored with radiation badges to show what and how much they are exposed to each day.

Radiation is only one category of occupational hazard. Under recent federal law, places where photographic chemicals and anesthetics are used may not employ pregnant women. But the risks run wider than that, and the safety nets are narrow. Some risks are so little known that they are discovered by chance—for example, when a group of workers talking together over coffee realize that they are all having trouble trying to have children.

For reproductive hazards alone, workers in these occupations are known to be at risk:

Graphic and plastic arts: exposure to solvents, paints, solder, clays, glazes, welding fumes, fumes from firing, poor ventilation. Heavy metals can damage kidney, liver, lungs, and the reproductive system.

Hospitals, medical laboratories , and other health care professions: a certain level of contact with radioactive materials or anesthetic gas adversely affects fertility in both men and women.

Nuclear power plants, atomic plants, and uranium mines: radiation can cause spontaneous abortion and genetic damage.

Metallurgy plants: exposure to copper, lead, arsenic, and cadmium can lead to sterility and birth defects. Metal grinders, lead smelter workers, lead storage-battery workers are at risk.

Radio and television manufacturing: exposure to solder fumes.

Chemical laboratories: exposure to solvents and other chemicals.

Plastics factories: exposure to polyvinyl chloride and other chemicals.

Hairdressing salons: chemicals, hair sprays and dyes, aerosol sprays, cosmetics, and other preparations can all have adverse reproductive effects.

Video display terminals (VDTs), widely used in various large businesses, were called into question when several Canadian VDT operators experienced miscarriages. Researchers at Mount Sinai Medical Center are conducting a survey of over ten thousand working women in the first major study to determine if there is a connection between the use of this equipment and problems in childbearing. Until the facts are in, it's wise to cover your own screen with a specially designed panel which cuts glare and also reduces very low frequency radiation. So far, VDTs have *not* been found to be a hazard to the fetus, but operators may experience neck pains or headaches from sitting in a fixed position for prolonged periods.

YOUR RIGHT TO KNOW

The difficulty in getting hard data about hazards has prompted some states to institute a Workers Right to Know program. At least eight states and six cities have adopted such bills, another twenty-five states have them under consideration.

Right to Know laws require manufacturers to inform employers about the risks of their substances, and for employers to pass this information on to employees—along with training in protective procedures.

With these new laws companies will face a choice—exclude both men and women from hazardous jobs, or clean up the workplace to eliminate reproductive risks. Both husband and wife should think about what they're exposed to at work, at home, and in communities. Studies on men are few, but wives of men who work in operating rooms and men who work with vinyl chloride are known to face an increased risk of miscarriage.

In 1981 John M. Peters and his colleagues at the University of Southern California School of Medicine compared the family histories of ninety-two children under age ten who had brain tumors with ninety-two matched controls. The mothers of children with brain tumors reported skin exposure to chemicals at three times greater frequency than did the control mothers, and the fathers were often employed in occupations involving solvents and in the aircraft industry. Exposure to chemical solvents by one or both parents was linked to brain tumors in their children, even though the parents exhibited no obvious negative effects.

WHAT YOU CAN DO

To make intelligent decisions about childbearing every working person needs to know the occupational risks he or she is facing. Describe to your physician the physical requirements of your job, as well as the chemicals, radiation, and/or fumes that you work with. Your obstetrician may suggest that you switch to another job before you become pregnant. Whatever your job, always follow any safety precautions that have been laid down, such as wearing a mask, respirator, or protective clothing.

If you suspect your working environment might be hazardous, talk to your employer or trade union. You may ask for the hazard to be removed or request better housekeeping—many occupational hazards can be remedied only by cleaning up the workplace.

Although management is supposed to provide a safe workplace, the real impetus usually comes from workers themselves. Recognition is the first step in eliminating hazards. First try to identify problems and then begin to build awareness about job conditions among fellow workers.

Learn about chemicals and other substances you work with. Ask management, or fellow workers in the supply department, to check the labels on the substances you work with; then write to the manufacturer and ask for the Material Safety Data Sheet.

If a chemical has been laboratory tested, you should be able to get more information from the safety department of your international union. The Committee for Occupational Safety and Health (COSH) is composed of thirty labor-based COSH groups around that country that advise workers about toxic effects and legal rights with respect to workplace chemicals.

You can also ask your employer to contact the local Occupational Safety and Health Administration (OSHA) office for the name of an industrial hygienist who will consult with your company free of charge. OSHA is listed in the government section of your local phone directory.

The National Institute for Occupational Safety and Health (NIOSH) will refer you or your employer to proper government agencies for occupational health concerns such as asbestos exposure and video display terminal use. Check local federal government listings for NIOSH.

Another good information source: Women's Occupational Health Resource Center, Columbia University School of Public Health, 21 Audubon Avenue, New York, N.Y. 10032

Identifying hazards in the workplace is definitely a pre-pregnancy task. By recognizing and eliminating any toxins there, you can help protect your fertility, as well as your baby's health.

Environmental hazards—whether they are personal habits such as smoking and drinking, drugs and stress, or whether they are toxins present in your workplace—are major causes of infertility and complications during pregnancy and childbirth. But they are not the only problems present in a modern society. Two other critical elements may compromise your reproductive capacity: venereal disease and contraceptives.

CHAPTER 9

PROTECTING YOUR
FUTURE FERTILITY

AN IMPORTANT COMPONENT of pre-pregnancy planning is making sure that when you are ready to have children you are able to conceive. The incidence of infertility has jumped from one couple in twelve ten years ago, to one couple in five today. At least half of these couples became infertile in adult life. Even if you know that you are fertile at this time of your life, there is a well-established risk that you may become infertile in the future. The elements conspiring against you include environmental hazards, which were discussed in the previous chapters, venereal disease, and contraceptives. Knowing how to cope with these invasive components of modern life will help ensure that when you are ready to have a family, your fertility will be intact.

VENEREAL DISEASE

Twenty years ago, blocked tubes, pelvic adhesions, and other obstructions accounted for only about 25 percent of infertility in women. Today, that figure has jumped to more than 40 percent. The major reason behind the soaring incidence of tubal blockage is infection of the pelvic cavity, called pelvic inflammatory disease (PID).

Such infections usually reach the pelvic cavity via sexual intercourse. Chlamydia is the most common sexually transmitted disease; gonorrhea is second. Chlamydia can invade and silently destroy the fallopian tubes within a few days. A woman may have had an undetected pelvic infection in her teens or twenties and never know that her reproductive organs were damaged until she finds herself unable to conceive in her thirties.

Not every bout of a sexually transmitted disease becomes PID, and not every episode of PID causes infertility. A woman who has one infection has a 15 percent chance of the infection invading the fallopian tubes and pelvic cavity. Once the infection goes that far, there is a 50 percent chance of infertility.

An army of white blood cells swarm over the foreign organisms in an effort to destroy the infection. As the white blood cells devour the bacteria they excrete a collagen protein that resembles steel mesh. This is scar tissue, which clogs and binds the narrow openings of the fallopian tubes, interfering with fertilization. Sometimes the tube is only partially blocked, setting up an obstacle course than can trap a fertilized egg and lead to tubal or ectopic pregnancy—a potentially life-threatening situation in which the fertilized egg begins to develop outside of the uterus. Early diagnosis and rapid treatment with proper antibiotics can halt the infection before it becomes PID. If the infection becomes full-blown PID, aggressive treatment can prevent massive damage, but even a remnant of scar tissue in the wrong place can interfere with conception.

With subsequent venereal infections the probability of damage increases, because the protective barriers guarding the reproductive organs have been worn away by previous invasions. The more sexual partners a woman has in her lifetime, the greater the odds of contracting a sexually transmitted disease. Although today, with the widespread incidence of venereal disease, even a single sexual encounter presents a substantial risk of infection. Further, a couple may have a silent infection without knowing it. They may be monogamous, yet unwittingly transmit the infection back and forth. Diagnosis and aggressive treatment of *both* partners is essential to protect fertility.

The worst thing about PID is that few symptoms may appear in the early stages of infection. As the disease progresses, pain is the main symptom—sharp sensations with pressure on the bladder and pain during intercourse; a pelvic infection may or may not be associated with fever. Sometimes, a slight blood-tinged discharge after intercourse is also present. Other possible symptoms: burning during urination; fever, chills, and vomiting; pain in the legs, back, and abdomen.

These symptoms are often confused with other conditions. Symptoms may worsen or they may subside. If they abate, the disease may be ignored, but a low-grade infection remains. It's not unusual for a woman who has had an undetected infection when she was younger to discover years later that she is unable to become pregnant because of damaging scars resulting from that infection. A ruptured appendix or other organs that become infected in childhood (bowel operations or hernias) can also cause tubal adhesions.

If PID is diagnosed accurately and proper treatment is begun immediately, the chances of preserving fertility dramatically increase. Chances are even better when a venereal disease is caught before it invades the pelvic cavity and turns into PID.

If you think you have been exposed to a venereal infection—don't wait for symptoms to appear. See your gynecologist immediately, and tell him or her why you have come; ask for a pelvic exam, a slide analysis *and* culture.

Full-blown infections will show up immediately on a slide test performed in the physician's office. If the slide analysis is negative, early infection may become apparent when bacteria are cultured and allowed to grow in the proper environment for twenty-four hours. If you feel certain you were exposed to disease, your physician may prescribe a protective course of antibiotics for you while you wait to learn the results of the culture.

Chlamydia

Gonorrhea used to be the most common cause of PID; about 25 percent of women with any form of gonorrhea will have significant tubal damage. However, recent studies show that most women with PID have several invading organisms present at the same time, and the most dangerous of all is the newly recognized organism called chlamydia. Although chlamydia has been known for centuries, it is a fragile organism and almost impossible to pinpoint. Today, thanks to new diagnostic tests, chlamydia is recognized as the most widespread of all sexually transmitted diseases, far surpassing gonorrhea as the leading cause of venereal disease in the United States.

Little attention was paid to chlamydia until researchers began to speculate that some unidentified, "nonspecific" organism was partly responsible for the high incidence of PID in infertile women. Finer diagnostic tests developed in the 1960s eventually were able to identify this elusive organism.

Chlamydia is more dangerous than any other invading organism because it can silently destroy the fallopian tubes within a few days without producing any symptoms at all. In fact, in 75 percent of cases no symptoms appear until PID is well advanced.

Chlamydia is equally destructive to men. Gonorrhea and other infections are not a significant cause of male infertility because they seldom reach the ductal system. The urethra, the only outside entrance into the male reproductive system, is comparatively long in men and as bacteria work their way along this tract, they are intermittently pushed back by streams of urine flushing out the passageway. Therefore, men are usually spared the devastating infections that destroy the reproductive organs of women. Further, gonorrhea is so easily recognized that men usually seek treatment when they first notice any unusual discharge, an early warning sign, from the penis.

Chlamydia, however, can reach the ductal system, causing inflammation and permanent scarring. It can also damage sperm. Typical symptoms of chlamydia in men are easily confused with those of gonorrhea but, unfortunately, the same penicillin-type drugs that easily eradicate gonorrhea have no effect on chlamydia. Only a tetracycline class of antibiotic can kill the organism, which means that correct diagnosis is imperative.

The real threat of any infection in a man is that it is easily transmitted to women, in whom it can cause sterility. Many men unwittingly transfer symptomless diseases such as chlamydia to women during sexual intercourse. Without treatment chlamydia remains in the system; a man or woman can harbor the disease for years without symptoms, passing it along to sexual partners. To prevent such transfers, fertility experts recommend that even mild, innocuous infections of the male reproductive tract be vigorously treated with antibiotics.

Danger to the Baby. A baby born to a mother with a chlamydia infection may become infected as it passes through the birth canal during labor. Chlamydia can cause eye infections (conjunctivitis) and pneumonia in newborns. Ideally every woman should be screened for chlamydia before becoming pregnant, but researchers say it is impossible to perform such screening on a widespread basis.

The diagnostic test for chlamydia, although vastly improved, is expensive and still requires special handling.

Prevention. Is there any solution to this epidemic which health experts admit is out of control and getting worse? If chlamydia and other organisms that cause pelvic infections present few symptoms, how can they be identified?

According to the conservative medical profession the spread of venereal disease is due to increased sexual permissiveness. The equation is: more sexual activity equals more venereal disease. More venereal disease means more pelvic infections, which lead to more infertility problems.

The general view is that the best way to halt the spread of venereal disease is for people to "behave right." This pervasive attitude has stymied research into venereal diseases. The same attitude that hampered the work of German bacteriologist Paul Ehrlich at the turn of the century hampers research into venereal disease today. Many physicians were against Ehrlich's development of the compound Salvarsan which specifically counteracted syphilis and other spirochetal infections because they felt that the possibility of contracting deadly syphilis prevented immoral sexual activity.

That same attitude holds true today. But the truth is that the epidemic is so widespread that you can contract chlamydia even if you have only one sexual partner in your lifetime. There are numerous instances of married couples passing the disease back and forth, with both being unaware that they have it. The problem may never be diagnosed, or it may eventually be discovered when one or the other partners proves infertile.

One young woman reported that she had severe bouts of pain for several years. Her doctor tested her for gonorrhea and found nothing. She was told that her stomach pains were probably stress-related. When she eventually had a complete fertility workup, which included a laparoscopy (an internal viewing of the pelvis), her reproductive organs were coated with scar tissue. The fertility specialist tested for chlamydia and found it; her husband also had the disease.

The solution to the chlamydia epidemic does not seem to be changing the behavior of the world at large. The solution is better diagnostic testing and better informed physicians who can make an accurate diagnosis and institute early treatment.

One new blood test (immunofluorescent) can now identify chlamydia in four hours. Some physicians routinely administer the test whenever their female patients come in for a routine checkup or Pap test. A vital part of the solution, however, is follow-up of an infected person's sexual contacts. It's estimated that one in ten college students has chlamydia. Yet because doctors are not required to report chlamydia to the public health authority, there is no systematic follow-up of contacts. As difficult as follow-up is, it seems a crucial element in the effort to bring the disease under control.

Herpes Virus

Herpes simplex, along with papovavirus or condyloma acuminatum (venereal warts), is a sexually transmitted virus. Unlike bacteria, viruses do not directly invade the reproductive tract to create scar tissue around internal organs. But they do seem to lead the way by altering the chemical balance within the vagina, so that bacteria have an easier invasion path. Such alterations of the vaginal fluids may also be lethal to sperm.

Viruses can also be dangerous to the fetus during pregnancy. Once begun, the herpes virus comes and goes in sporadic outbreaks of genital lesions that may vary from a slight red bump to clusters of blisters. The first infection is usually more virulent than recurrent episodes: if a woman gets herpes for the first time during the early weeks of pregnancy, she has a 25 percent greater chance of spontaneous abortion than an unaffected woman.

Herpes may also be passed on to the baby during vaginal delivery, but only if the disease is active when the child passes through the birth canal. If the baby does contract the disease—the odds are 50–50—it is likely to suffer brain damage, blindness, and possibly death. However, if the virus is dormant at the time of labor vaginal delivery is safe. If a pregnant woman knows she has herpes, her physician will watch her carefully and take routine blood tests. If signs of herpes appear the obstetrician will schedule a cesarean delivery. But since herpes can erupt suddenly without notice, some physicians routinely recommend cesarean delivery for any woman who has a history of herpes virus.

Other Causes of Scarring

Events other than infections can cause scarring of reproductive organs. A ruptured appendix or a ruptured ovarian cyst that bleeds into the pelvic cavity often causes scarring. Any surgery performed within the pelvic cavity can also build scar tissue around reproductive organs. If you must have abdominal surgery, select a surgeon who uses refined microsurgical techniques. Superior surgical technique can reduce internal scarring. For unknown reasons, however, any surgery, no matter how slight, will create rubbery scar tissue in some women. At the other extreme, some women who have had severe infections or surgical complications will not develop any scar tissue at all. Both extremes are exceptions; in general, the amount of scar tissue corresponds to the extent of the surgery or infection.

CONTRACEPTIVES

Can the contraceptive you use today compromise your fertility tomorrow? The answer may be yes. It's important that couples who wish to protect their fertility for future pregnancies pay close attention to the type of contraceptives they choose. For example, certain contraceptives can increase—or diminish—the risk of contracting pelvic inflammatory infection.

The diaphragm and condom, which block the entry of sperm into the cervix, also help block bacteria. The birth control pill, which sustains a tough cervical mucus all month long, also helps guard against some, but not all, infectious organisms.

By contrast, the IUD leaves a clear runway for bacteria-laden sperm to travel. Women using an IUD who have never had a baby are seven to ten times more likely to develop PID than a woman who uses other forms of birth control.

You may decide to change the contraceptive you use several months before you try to become pregnant. Your choice of contraceptive depends on your age, your health, your present fertility status, and your lifestyle. The best contraceptive is usually one that offers the most protection with the fewest side effects. So far, no contraceptive is ideal; each comes with its own set of advantages and disadvantages: some of the more effective ones, like the pill and the IUD, may produce side effects. The safer barrier methods—condoms and diaphragms—have other drawbacks. And the spermicides have a relatively high failure rate.

Oral Contraceptives

For various reasons most fertility experts recommend that a woman stop taking the birth control pill at least three months *before she tries* to become pregnant. Long-term use of the pill, coupled with poor diet, can increase your risk of vitamin deficiency. The vitamins are naturally replenished within two to three months after you stop using the pill.

However, the major problem, as far as future fertility is concerned, is that after a woman stops taking the pill it may take three or four months for ovulation to resume. And about 20 percent of women who take the pill need as long as a year to regain their fertility. This can be a serious problem for a woman who has delayed pregnancy until her mid-thirties, when her fertility is in decline. A small percentage of women never regain their fertility after taking the pill. Because of this time factor it is recommended that women planning to delay childbirth discontinue the pill by age thirty and switch to another form of birth control.

Studies suggest that length of use of the pill does not affect future fertility, but consistency of use does. A woman who goes on and off the pill will have more trouble regaining regular ovulation than a woman who consistently uses the pill.

The pre-pill menstrual cycle is another factor. Women who had regular cycles before they started taking the pill usually recover normal ovulation and menstrual function quickly after stopping. Those who had erratic cycles when they started the pill take the longest to recoup.

Of all the contraceptives available, only the pill prevents the union of sperm and egg by stopping egg production, which accounts for its remarkable success rate.

The pill acts by jamming a wrench into the cyclical hormonal flow between the brain and the ovaries that governs ovulation. The hormonal axis shuts down, and the pill takes over, parceling out a steady supply of hormones all month long. Eggs do not develop in the ovaries and therefore are not released into the fallopian tubes.

The chances of becoming pregnant on the pill are about 1 percent. In these cases the chemical blockade is not strong enough to hold back the hormonal axis. Should you become pregnant while on the pill, there may be some danger that the progesterone in the pill might adversely affect the early development of the fetal organs. However, several studies exploring this hypothesis showed that birth defects among pregnant women who had been exposed to progesterone were no higher than those in the unexposed group. Until the controversy is settled, however, it is another good reason to wait three months after stopping the pill before trying to become pregnant. In the interval, the best form of contraceptive is the condom or diaphragm.

One advantage of the pill is that women are protected against some infections because the mucus barrier that guards the cervix remains thick and inpenetrable all month long, hence preventing the transmission of disease during sexual intercourse. Unfortunately, the most insidious of venereal infections, chlamydia, seems able to get past this barrier and invade the pelvic cavity. New research from the Centers for Disease Control in Atlanta shows that the steroids in birth control pills alter vaginal pH, creating a climate conducive to chlamydia growth.

In other ways, however, the modern low-dose contraceptive pill, which combines estrogen with progesterone, appears safe and effective for most younger women. Every woman taking the pill should be aware of the risk of chlamydia infection and should also be screened by her doctor twice a year for any sign of high blood pressure, heart disease, or other problems.

The pill becomes less safe after age thirty. Women between thirty and thirty-five can continue to use the pill unless they are obese, smoke cigarettes, or have preexisting diseases. After age thirty-five, side effects of the pill become more dangerous for all women, regardless of their weight or blood pressure or whether they smoke.

You should not use birth control pills at any age if you have any of the following conditions: high blood pressure, impaired liver function; thrombophlebitis (blood clots), stroke, or coronary artery disease; severe migraine headaches; breast cancer; sickle-cell anemia.

Intrauterine Devices
After the birth control pill, the IUD is the most effective method of reversible contraception. It has two advantages over the pill: the IUD allows the body to go through its natural hormonal changes every month, and it is permanent until removed. The disadvantage is that an IUD offers no protection against the transmission of vene-

real disease and, in fact, encourages many different kinds of infections that can lead to infertility.

An IUD is a small coil placed in the uterus. Surprisingly, no one knows exactly how the IUD works. Some scientists contend that the device acts as a barrier between sperm and egg. Others say that the IUD causes the lining of the uterus and fallopian tubes to become so inflamed that the egg cannot be fertilized or, if it is fertilized, it cannot implant in the uterus.

The chronic irritation creates an ideal surface for infection to take hold. And the strings that descend into the vagina (present in some IUDs) can act as a wick for bacteria to enter the uterus. It is estimated that women using IUDs have two to three times as much chance of developing pelvic infections as those using other contraceptives or no birth control at all.

Sometimes an IUD will penetrate the wall of the uterus and pass into the abdomen. This poses no immediate physical danger, but it can have serious consequences for fertility. The omentum, a fatty curtain of tissue that hangs from the upper portion of the colon, engulfs the puncture in an effort to stop the spread of infection. The puncture heals, unnoticed. Evidence of the wound may show up years later when the woman is infertile because the omentum is stuck to the surface of the uterus and tubes.

IUDs come in many sizes and shapes. Risk is lowest among users of copper-coated IUDs. Infections seem to occur more often in women who have never had a child because the uterus is smaller and more easily irritated by the device. Therefore, in terms of protecting your future fertility, the IUD is most suitable for women who have only one sexual partner (less risk of venereal disease) and those who have already had children. Young women postponing childbirth or women planning their first child would be better off with a different kind of contraceptive.

If you do use an IUD, you can become pregnant as soon as it is removed. Occasionally a woman will become pregnant with the IUD in place. If this happens to you, you have a 50 percent risk of spontaneous abortion. There is an equal chance of carrying the child safely to term without removal of the device. However, most physicians recommend that the IUD be removed as soon as possible after a pregnancy is detected, to avoid life-threatening complications such as septicemia, septic shock, and septic abortion.

Recently, G. D. Searle & Company announced that it was discontinuing the sale of its two intrauterine contraceptive devices in the United States. The company's decision was due to increasing costs of product-liability litigation and insurance. With Searle's withdrawal, the IUD is no longer available in this country. However, the FDA still approves the use of IUDs. Women who are currently using IUDs are not required to have them removed, but the devices should not be left in place for more than three years.

Spermicides

Spermicides have received negative press lately for two reasons: high failure rate (thirty out of a hundred women become pregnant when using spermicides alone). Second, a higher than usual number of late miscarriages and birth defects have been reported in women who accidentally conceive while using a spermicide, supposedly because the spermicide damages the DNA of the sperm. However, new research suggests that such abnormalities were caused by other factors and that spermicides are relatively safe.

Despite these conflicting reports, spermicides have some outstanding advantages. They can be purchased without a doctor's prescription; they may offer some protection against gonorrhea, chlamydia, and the herpes virus; and they do not appear to affect future fertility.

Spermicides, which are marketed as foams, creams, jellies, foaming tablets, and suppositories, contain a sperm-killing detergent, nonoxynol-9, which coats the sperm and chokes off their oxygen supply. They also contain a bulky substance that partially blocks the cervix and helps prevent any surviving sperm from entering the uterus.

The high failure rate associated with spermicides is due partly to improper use. Creams and jellies, which contain less spermicide and fail to coat the cervix or vagina evenly, should be used with a diaphragm. The foam, foaming tablets, and suppositories can be used alone. When a spermicide is combined with a condom or a diaphragm it provides excellent protection against pregnancy; this combination may be the safest, most effective method of birth control.

Fertility is restored as soon as a woman stops using a spermicide. Until the controversy about miscarriage and birth defects is resolved, couples should stop using spermicides a month or so before the woman tries to become pregnant and use only a condom in the interval.

The Sponge

The polyurethane sponge acts by blocking the cervix, absorbing sperm, and coating them with nonoxynol-9. The advantage of the sponge over foams and other forms of spermicides is that each sponge provides twenty-four-hour protection, so that sexual relations do not have to be interrupted in order to reapply a contraceptive. Sponges are available over the counter without prescription.

However, the sponge, which is confined to one specific area, may prevent only cervical infections; it will not prevent vaginal infections and may, in fact, encourage them by blocking natural cervical secretions. Several cases of septic shock syndrome have been associated with the sponge. The other disadvantages are the same as those associated with all spermicides, mainly a relatively high failure rate and suspected danger of increased birth defects if a woman accidentally becomes pregnant while using the contraceptive.

Women who use spermicide-type contraceptives should be alert for further reports regarding possible side effects.

Barrier Devices

Barrier devices such as the diaphragm and condom are safe and effective, protecting against both pregnancy and venereal disease. Before the birth control pill became available, these devices were the most widely used contraceptives in the world. Today they have become popular again, largely because they help reduce the spread of venereal infection and don't have the side effects associated with new contraceptives.

The problem with barrier devices is that, compared to the pill, they are awkward and sometimes inconvenient to use. Even though condoms fit like skin, many men feel that they interfere with sexual pleasure.

The Diaphragm. A diaphragm is a soft latex cup that a woman fills with spermicidal jelly or cream and inserts over the cervix. It offers protection against cervical infections caused by gonorrhea, chlamydia, and trichomonas. However, the diaphragm protects against vaginal infections only if you follow its insertion with an application of spermicidal foam.

A diaphragm must be fitted by a physician or nurse; and the fit checked every six months. Failure rates range from 6 to 29 percent. Improper use and failure to check for pin-size holes contribute to the high variation in failure rates.

Used properly, the diaphragm offers protection and has no affect on future fertility. Diaphragms seem to work best for older women who are well motivated to use contraception and who have one sexual partner. Younger women, and women who have some conflict about using a contraceptive, seem to have a higher failure rate. The side effects with the diaphragm are the same as those related to spermicides.

The diaphragm is especially recommended for women coming off the pill who are waiting for their normal hormonal cycle to resume before becoming pregnant.

The Cervical Cap. The cervical cap, which can be left in place for several days at a time, is like a semipermanent diaphragm. Several versions of the device are now being tested in the United States, including a molded plastic model which can stay in place for several months. Ultimately this experimental cap may be the answer for women who want the safety of the diaphragm plus the convenience of an IUD or birth control pill. The worry is that the cap may encourage the growth of some infections by blocking the flow of natural secretions that normally cleanse the vagina.

The Condom. The condom, one of the oldest forms of birth control, is the world's most widely used contraceptive and the single most important guard against sexually transmitted disease. By preventing semen, a rich culture medium, from spilling into the vagina, a condom discourages bacterial growth. It also acts as a shield between the penis and vagina, and it protects against the transmission of all types of organisms. There is some question whether or not the herpes virus can pass through the pores of a condom. (Most doctors say it does.) But the condom protects against chlamydia, gonorrhea, Trichomonas, *Candida, Hemophilus vaginalis,* and, to some extent, syphilis and venereal warts.

When a man uses a condom and his partner uses a spermicide, the combination is a highly effective contraceptive. The failure rate, which ranges from 5 to 25 percent, is related to improper use.

A condom is the safest contraceptive to use in the interval in which you prepare to become pregnant.

Coitus Interruptus

Interruption of sexual intercourse to prevent pregnancy is the least effective of all contraceptive methods. For the method to work a man must withdraw from intercourse completely before he has ejaculated even a single drop of semen. (The first portion of the ejaculate is the most potent, containing 80 percent of the sperm.) Even sperm deposited on the outer lips of the vagina can make their way up the vaginal canal and through the cervix.

The chances of accomplishing complete, early withdrawal on a regular basis are virtually nil; therefore, the greatest risk that accompanies coitus interruptus is pregnancy. Nor does it offer protection against most venereal diseases.

The Rhythm Method

The idea of the rhythm method is to abstain from sexual intercourse on the days you are ovulating. The tricky part of this method is to know *when* ovulation occurs. The temperature chart and mucus method used to determine your most fertile days can be used conversely for contraception (see Chapter 6).

The safest way to use the chart is to abstain from intercourse for the first half of your menstrual cycle until three days after the shift in temperature occurs. The failure rate using this method is between 3.0 and 6.6 percent. But it means avoiding sexual intercourse for two weeks out of every month.

A woman who does not take her temperature, but goes strictly by her calendar, would abstain from intercourse for about ten days in the middle of her menstrual cycle, roughly between days nine and nineteen of a twenty-eight-day cycle. The failure rate with this method, however, is considerably higher, between 7 and 20 percent.

Abstinence methods require vigilance, and it's easy to make a mistake. They work best for young women with regular menstrual cycles. (As a woman grows older and her ovulation pattern becomes more erratic, it's more difficult to predict when the egg will be released from an ovary.)

The rhythm method is free of chemical side effects, but it obviously does not protect against the transmission of disease. There is also a certain amount of stress involved. The best candidates for this form of birth control are couples determined to avoid other forms of contraceptives—or unconcerned about an accidental pregnancy. In other words, if you've just come off a contraceptive and want to wait a while before becoming pregnant, or if you have the attitude "if it happens, it happens," then rhythm is feasible.

Abortion
For several reasons, not least among them emotional stress, abortion cannot be considered a standard form of contraception. However, a woman who elects to have an abortion to terminate an unwanted pregnancy is not usually risking her future fertility. Voluntary abortion today is a choice governed by personal feelings rather than by health risks. Women who have a properly performed, early abortion usually suffer no physical complications, and their fertility is not compromised. Occasional complications may arise from unskilled surgical technique, or when the abortion is performed during the more advanced stages of pregnancy. The earlier the abortion is performed, the less risk of complications. Should infection arise following an abortion, an uncommon event with legal abortions, the reproductive organs may become scarred and result in infertility.

Sterilization
A vasectomy for a man or tubal ligation for a woman is permanent sterilization. Much has been made of the news that a handful of surgical wizards can restore fertility by reconnecting the vasa deferentia in men, or the fallopian tubes in women, but these expensive, complicated reversals are successful only about 60 percent of the time.

Any man or woman considering sterilization as a form of birth control should make certain that he or she does not want children in the future. Reversals are most often requested when a divorced or widowed person wants to start a second family. In these instances it may be worth it to try for a reversal.

The Future
A new technique to temporarily block a woman's fallopian tubes with removable silicone implants is under investigation. A surgeon uses a long slender telescope, called a hysteroscope, to insert foam-

ing silicone through the cervix and into the uterus. Once the tubes are located, the silicone is pushed in; the foam hardens into a small plug inside the tubes. The idea is that the plugs can be removed later, and fertility will be intact.

There are still numerous problems with the implants, and reversibility has not been proved. However, if the technique is perfected, it may revolutionize contraception. The implants have no side effects, create no chemical changes within the body, and leave both partners free from concern about contraception. They will not, however, offer any protection against venereal disease.

Many more contraceptives are under investigation today, including modified birth control pills, antipregnancy vaccines, and the erstwhile male contraceptive. While all of these are interesting, much more research is needed before they might be tested on a wide scale.

The most promising—and most imminent—is Norplant, a thin cluster of six inch-long rods implanted under a woman's arm. Norplant releases a constant flow of low-dosage progesterone for up to five years, with a failure rate of less than 1 percent. The implants involve a minor surgical procedure performed in five to ten minutes in a doctor's office. Norplant is presently in use in fourteen countries, but after more than fifteen years of testing it has not yet been approved for use in the United States.

Another experimental drug—known only by its identifying number RV486—is sometimes called abortion without surgery. The drug blocks the delivery of progesterone to the uterus; because the endometrial lining of the uterus cannot thicken properly without progesterone, a fertilized ovum cannot implant. Without progesterone, the endometrium breaks up and discharges as a regular menstrual period.

As far as male contraceptives go, the Chinese continue to work on a male pill, but its availability appears to be at least ten years away.

Infertility is a rising epidemic in the United States and in many instances can be prevented. By recognizing and correcting the dangers—present in the environment, in contraceptives, and in the transmission of disease—women and men can do much to protect their health and future fertility. Knowing the hazards that exist, recognizing symptoms of disease, and seeking early medical advice will let you sidestep many of the otherwise devastating effects. These are preventive measures to help ensure that when you are ready to become pregnant your fertility will be intact. But there are also constructive steps that you can take to counteract some of the negative effects of environmental hazards and to *enhance* future pregnancies. These steps involve maximizing nutrition and general fitness. The following two chapters offer the first diet and exercise plans ever devised exclusively for women who wish to condition their bodies and meet their special needs for pregnancy before they conceive.

CHAPTER 10

THE PRE-PREGNANCY DIET

MOST OF US CONSIDERING pregnancy don't know how to prepare our bodies before conception occurs. We only begin to read books about nutrition several weeks or months after becoming pregnant. It's clear that poor nutrition increases the risk of producing an abnormal baby, but we often don't realize that the risk is greatest for women who are already poorly nourished when they conceive.

Four factors influence the health and size of the baby: your, the mother's, nutritional status; how long the child remains in the uterus; the amount of weight you gain during pregnancy; and how much you weigh *before* pregnancy.

Studies by Dr. Richard L. Naeye of Hershey Medical Center in Hershey, Pennsylvania, studied the relationship of the mother's pre-pregnancy weight to the survival of the baby in 53,518 pregnancies. He found that a woman who starts out underweight is more likely to deliver prematurely or deliver a baby who is dangerously small, even if she gains weight normally during pregnancy. And a woman who is obese to start with is more likely to develop serious pregnancy complications and to encounter difficulties in delivery that could jeopardize both the baby and mother.

Weight, however, is only one issue. Certain nutrients critical for pregnancy are typically lacking in the average woman's daily diet. By nutritionally preparing your body in advance, the embryo has all the advantages of optimum nutrition from the moment you become pregnant.

Another reason to beef up your store of pre-pregnancy nutrients: in the first several weeks following conception you may feel too sick to eat—if you are properly nourished before pregnancy your body will carry you through these early days without endangering the embryo.

A quality diet provides all the nutrients you need to help you have a healthy pregnancy and a healthy baby. It will also keep your immune system working properly, which will enable you to resist infection better. And, to some extent, a proper diet also helps protect against the harmful effects of environmental toxins and pollutants.

With the current emphasis on good nutrition, it's easy to assume that if you eat three square meals a day you must be getting enough of the nutrients you need. But, in term of a future pregnancy, you can eat plenty and still be malnourished.

The purpose of the Pre-Pregnancy Diet is twofold. The first benefit is to boost your body's nutritional status to an optimum level in preparation for a quality pregnancy. Certain specific vitamins and minerals, for example, can be stored by the body before conception, ready to be used the moment pregnancy places new demands on the body. The second benefit is to cleanse your system. If you were a smoker, used drugs, or consumed alcohol, the Pre-Pregnancy Diet offers a "detox" period to clear you body of harmful residues. This diet has been designed by Susan D. Shaw, noted nutritionist and environmental health consultant in New York City. For maximum effect, begin the program at least three months before you plan to conceive.

THE PRE-PREGNANCY DIET

The Pre-Pregnancy Diet contains a variety of foods from the basic food groups, with certain nutrients emphasized: protein, calcium, magnesium, vitamins C and E, iron, and the B complex vitamins, especially folic acid. These are the nutrients especially important for pregnancy.

Protein

Adequate amounts of high-quality protein will keep your muscles, organs, and other tissues in good repair and maintain the proper levels of hormones, blood cells, and enzymes in your body as you prepare for pregnancy. You will need extra protein to form healthy new tissue as you go into pregnancy.

High-quality protein means a "complete" protein that contains all eight essential amino acids (eggs, muscle meats, or fish). Body tissue cannot be built from the incomplete proteins found in most vegetables unless they are properly combined. You should not count on processed foods, or fried or "fast" foods to supply high-quality protein because their basic chemical structure is adulterated. (There is evidence that many fried or fast foods contain fats that have rancidified and may have cancer-causing effects.)

Calcium

Extra stores of calcium in the mother's body are crucial for the development of the baby's bones and tooth buds. It's recently been shown that increased calcium intake before and during pregnancy helps reduce the complications of toxemia during pregnancy, including elevated blood pressure, fluid retention, and protein spill into the urine. But calcium is something many women are lacking when they enter pregnancy. Further, refined sugars, alcohol, and caffeine cause large quantities of calcium and magnesium to be excreted in the urine.

You can help build stores of calcium by eliminating sugars, alcohol, and caffeine and by increasing your consumption of skim milk, yogurt, and other dairy products. Calcium is also found in dark green leafy vegetables, sesame seeds, almonds, and canned salmon (if bones are eaten). Susan Shaw notes that magnesium is vital to help the body absorb calcium. In fact, a magnesium-rich diet can help correct calcium-deficiency diseases. Nuts, whole grains, and all varieties of beans and peas are rich in magnesium, as are dark green leafy vegetables and seafoods.

Calcium is one of the five important pre-pregnancy vitamin/minerals that may need supplementation because it's almost impossible to get adequate calcium from food without going overboard on dairy products, which are high in calories and fat. In one recent study a supplement of 440 milligrams/day of calcium reduced the incidence of toxemia in one group of pregnant women from 14.6 to 4.8 percent. Going into pregnancy, you're looking for a total calcium consumption of 1,200–2,000 mg/day. A quart of milk supplies about

1,200 mg. Add 6 oz. of cheese for another 800 mg. (See the calcium chart.)

The B Complex Vitamins

Your need for two B complex vitamins—vitamin B_{12} and folic acid—doubles when you are pregnant, and it's a good idea to get started on building these nutrients before pregnancy. Too little folic acid is one of the most common deficiencies in pregnant women. These two vitamins work together to promote the formation of healthy red blood cells in the mother and DNA production in the fetus. Good sources of folic acid are dark green vegetables, asparagus, legumes (especially lima beans), whole grains, nuts, salmon, and lean meats. Vitamin B_{12} is found naturally in fish, organ meats, egg yolks, and cheese. Both of these vitamins often need to be supplemented during pregnancy.

If you've been taking oral contraceptives for several years, you will also need extra Vitamin B_6, folic acid, and zinc.

Iron

Few women start pregnancy with enough iron stored in their bodies. Iron is critical because your blood volume will double during pregnancy. It's difficult to get enough iron because only 10 percent of the iron taken in supplements or in foods is actually taken up by the body.

Iron-rich foods include all lean meats, dark green vegetables (especially parsley and kale), beets and beet greens, dried fruits (for example, apricots, prunes, or figs), egg yolks, shellfish, molasses, and whole grains. Organ meats, such as liver, heart, and kidney, are also rich in iron, although it's important to make sure these come from organic sources that are free from chemicals. Legumes (beans and peas) provide dietary iron, but recent studies suggest that eating large quantities of legumes such as soybeans is not an effective way to increase iron stores in the body.

If you are anemic, Susan Shaw suggests that the body's iron stores be replenished by eating plenty of iron-rich foods, along with high-quality protein, in the months before pregnancy. *Iron supplements are not recommended unless absolutely necessary.* Do not take iron supplements without first consulting your physician. Anemia can be caused by a

RELATIONSHIP OF CALCIUM TO
CALORIES, FATS, AND PROTEIN

Dairy Products

	Calcium (mg)	Calories	Protein (gr)	Fats (gr)
Whole milk, 32 oz.	1,140	660	32	40
Skim milk, 32 oz.	1,192	360	36	trace
Buttermilk, cultured, 8 oz.	298	127	9	5
Yogurt, part skim milk, 8 oz.	295	120	8	4
Cream, light or half & half, 4 oz.	130	170	4	15
Cream, heavy, 4 oz.	82	430	2	47
Cottage cheese, 8 oz.	207	240	30	11
nonfat cottage cheese, 8 oz.	202	195	38	trace
Cheddar cheese, 4 oz.	435	226	14	19
Cream cheese, 1 oz.	18	105	2	11
Roquefort cheese, 1 oz.	122	105	6	9
Swiss cheese, 1 oz.	270	105	7	8

Other Calcium Sources

Dark greens (kale, spinach), 8 oz.	130	45	4	1
Almonds, 4 oz.	163	425	13	38
Sesame seeds, 4 oz.	580	280	9	24
Salmon, canned (w/bones), 3 oz.	160	120	17	5
Sardines, canned (w/bones), 3 oz.	367	180	22	9

NOTE: Calcium is more readily absorbed from whole milk than skim milk products because the presence of some fat aids absorption. However, even if milk and dairy products are eaten frequently, it is difficult to get an adequate supply of calcium unless calcium supplements are taken.

deficiency of many nutrients other than iron, including folic acid, B_{12}, B_6, and vitamin E.

Vitamin C

Proper amounts of vitamin C are needed both before and during pregnancy. Research has established that vitamin C has important effects on the vitality of the developing child, as well as on the immune system of a pregnant woman. Vitamin C is found naturally in a wide variety of fruits and vegetables. Citrus fruits, papaya, mango, guava, cantaloupe, broccoli, brussels sprouts, green and red peppers, parsley, and strawberries are all good sources of vitamin C.

Cigarette smoking plays havoc with your body's absorption of vitamin C. Smoking one cigarette, for example, is known to deplete 100 mg of vitamin C. Throughout this book we have emphasized the need to stop smoking during pregnancy, and you cannot counteract the harmful effects of smoking by taking vitamin C supplements. But if you are in the process of quitting you may need to add some extra vitamin C to your diet now.

Vitamin C supplements in low to moderate levels—between 200–1,000 mg daily—appear safe before and during pregnancy. Very high levels, in the thousands of milligrams a day, are not recommended because they are thought to create a transient vitamin dependency in the fetus.

Vitamin E

Vitamin E is the only fat-soluble vitamin needed in increased amounts going into pregnancy. There is evidence that vitamin E helps promote fertility in both sexes, and the need for this vitamin doubles during pregnancy, particularly during the second trimester. Vitamin E is found in meat, fish, grains, liver, yeast, nuts, and the oils of wheat germ, soybeans, cottonseed, and corn.

Zinc

Zinc deprivation in humans has been associated with reduced fertility in women, retarded growth of the fetus, abnormal fetal development, and prolonged labor.

Zinc-rich foods include oysters, herring, whole grains, liver, lamb, beef, poultry, nuts, brown rice, peas, peanuts, milk, and eggs. Zinc absorption is enhanced by adequate levels of iron, vitamin B_6, and dietary tryptophan, an amino acid found in lean meats, fish, eggs, and dairy products.

What about Vitamin and Mineral Supplements?

Vitamins and minerals, although needed in only small amounts, are necessary to promote growth, reproduction, and maintenance of cell life. While a well-balanced diet provides most vitamins and minerals, there is clear evidence that increasing your intake of certain nutrients, such as calcium, folic acid, and other B vitamins, to above-dietary levels can be beneficial to your pregnancy.

In one study, women who had previously given birth to one or more babies with a neural tube defect were given a vitamin/mineral supplement for at least four weeks before their next conception, and for the first eight weeks of pregnancy. The vitamin group was found to be seven times *less* likely to have another handicapped baby than was a control group of women who did not take the supplement. The vitamin deficiency most clearly associated with this problem is folic acid.

Even with an adequate diet, nutrients may be destroyed in the environment or in the body, may be improperly absorbed into the blood, or may be excreted too hastily as a result of many complex factors. Even if you begin an optimal diet now, if your diet has been deficient in the past, supplements may be needed to help you more quickly establish good nutritional status.

Vitamins are divided into two categories: water-soluble and fat-soluble. It's important to know the difference between the two groups.

Fat-soluble vitamins—A, D, E, and K—are stored by the body, which means they can accumulate and become toxic if you ingest too much. Your need for the fat-soluble vitamins does not usually increase in pregnancy and you can get adequate levels of these vitamins with a high-quality diet. In fact, an excess of fat-soluble vitamins may have adverse effects on the mother and developing fetus, and supplements should not be taken unless your physician recommends them for a specific condition. The one exception is vitamin E supplementation, which can benefit you.

Water-soluble vitamins—C and the B vitamins—are a different story. These vitamins are rapidly absorbed and rapidly excreted. Rapid excretion in the urine means that they have to be replenished

COMPLETE PRE-PREGNANCY NUTRITION PROGRAM
Total of All Nutrients Required from All Sources

(Daily, from diet and supplements combined)

Calories	1,500–2,500
Protein	75–120 gr
Fluids	3–5 pt.
Salt	6–8 gr
Essential fats	3–10 gr
	(2 tbs of cold-pressed veg oil)

Vitamins

A	5,000–20,000 IU
D	400–800 IU
E	100–400 IU
C	200–1,000 mg
B_1	5–100 mg
B_2	5–100 mg
B_3	5–100 mg
B_6	5–100 mg
B_{12}	5–200 mg
folic acid	800–2,000 mcg
pantothenic acid	50–200 mg
biotin	50–100 mcg

Minerals

calcium	1,200–2,000 mg
magnesium	600–1,000 mg
phosphorus	1,400–1,800 mg
iron	20–60 mg
copper	2–5 mg
zinc	20–40 mg
choline	100–1,000 mg
inositol	100–1,000 mg
PABA	5–100 mg
manganese	5–10 mg
chromium	50–100 mcg
selenium	100–200 mcg
iodine	200–500 mg

regularly, and it also means that it's hard to overdose on them (although it's possible). The most recent research shows that a woman's need for the water-soluble vitamins increases throughout pregnancy.

Looking at the total picture, even when you follow a good pre-pregnancy diet program, the evidence suggests that supplements can help. "Pre-pregnancy is a good time to optimize," says Shaw. "Calcium, magnesium, and the other important vitamins—the B complex vitamins, especially folic acid and B_{12}, and vitamin C—these are the same supplements that can be continued at safe levels through pregnancy." She cautions against megadoses because excess quantities of some vitamins and minerals can be just as damaging as deficiencies of them.

The key to optimizing before pregnancy is combining a nutrient-rich diet with a supplement program based on your own unique needs. However, Susan Shaw has devised the following moderate supplement plan, within prudent ranges of the USRDA, which most women can safely follow before becoming pregnant. (See the supplement chart). These same supplements can often be continued throughout pregnancy, but because each woman's needs are different, always consult your obstetrician before taking supplements during pregnancy.

Starting Your Diet
The Pre-Pregnancy Diet offers you an opportunity to select from a wide variety of high-quality nutrients. A good pre-pregnancy regimen means an intake of 1,500 to 2,500 calories per day, including three to five pints of water and other fluids. The idea is to eat a variety of the foods you like and to adjust the caloric content to fit your individual needs.

For example, if you exercise a lot, if you are large-framed, or if you are underweight, make sure your total calories per day are in the upper range. If you are small-framed, or if you are slightly overweight, your total daily calories should be in the lower range. (If you don't presently exercise, now is a good time to start.) There is clear evidence that exercising increases your need for antioxidant nutrients. Make sure to take supplements of the antioxidant vitamins C and E. If you perform aerobic exercise several times a week, take the supplement in the upper range recommended.

RECOMMENDED PRE-PREGNANCY SUPPLEMENTS

	Supplement Range
Vitamin E	
(d-alpha tocopherol acetate)	100–400 IU
Vitamin C	200–1,000 mg
Vitamn B complex*	
B_1 (thiamine)	5–50 mg
B_2 (riboflavin)	5–50 mg
B_3 (niacinamide)	5–50 mg
B_5 (pantothenic acid)	10–100 mg
B_6 (pyridoxine)	5–100 mg
B_{12} (cobalamin)	5–50 mcg
Folic acid	800–2,000 mcg
Biotin	10–50 mcg
Choline	10–100 mg
Inositol	10–100 mg
PABA	10–50 mg
Calcium	800–1,200 mg
carbonate (oyster shell), lactate or orotate; chelated is all right, but less calcium per mg is absorbed by the body)	
Magnesium	400–600 mg

NOTE: Unless specifically formulated, multivitamins are *not* recommended going into pregnancy because they usually contain iron salts and fat-soluble vitamins that should not be taken in a supplementary form. Likewise, the one-a-day prenatal prescription supplements for pregnant women are usually inadequate sources of key nutrients, notably folic acid.

* The B vitamins do not need to be taken separately. A single good B complex vitamin should contain all of the necessary B vitamins in adequate amounts. Compare labels carefully. Yeast-free vitamins are recommended for people with allergies.

By choosing a wide variety of foods from the basic categories that follow, you will begin to store all of the pregnancy nutrients in advance. Make sure to choose unrefined and unprocessed foods which ensure optimum nutrient content. If you recognize any nutrient previously missing from your diet, for example, iron or folic acid, make sure to include ample amounts in your pre-pregnancy program. Here are the basics.

Protein foods—Three to Four Servings a Day

High-quality protein should be at the level of 75 to 120 grams per day, which is equivalent to a total of 10 to 16 ounces of lean meats, fish, poultry, or cheese.

High-quality protein should be 20 to 30 percent of the calories in your pre-pregnancy diet. Eggs are an excellent source of protein and are also packed with many different nutrients because they are intended to contain everything chicks need to develop.

Protein foods, particularly animal protein, need to be spaced or "rotated" in your diet to ensure balance and variety. Also some of these foods (such as cow's milk, beef, or eggs, as well as grains and oats) tend to cause allergies in some people. For those who are allergic, this problem can be greatly diminished by rotating proteins and other allergenic foods.

Milk, yogurt (preferably a live-culture brand that is natural and unsweetened), cottage cheese, and hard and soft cheeses fall into the protein group. Avoid processed cheese and cheese spreads, which usually contain additives. Dairy products are the primary source of calcium.

Fish, preferably cooked, of all varieties offers high-quality protein. Oily fish—sardines, salmon, bluefish, or tuna—are an excellent source of essential fatty acids and other nutrients and should be included in the diet. However, tuna and swordfish contain appreciable amounts of mercury, a toxic metal that can damage the nervous system and should be eaten only in limited quantities. Raw fish (sushi) is another source of mercury and various antinutrients and should also be limited.

Lean muscle meats, such as veal and chicken (without the skin), offer high-quality protein and low fat content. Liver is high in iron and other valuable vitamins and minerals, but seek out organic (chemical-free) organ meats.

Legumes, such as peas, beans, and lentils, bean sprouts, and soy products (tofu, miso, and so on) are good sources of vegetable protein, as are nuts and seeds (sunflower, sesame, and pumpkin). Whole grains also supply appreciable amounts of vegetable protein. However, except for yeast, soybeans, sprouts, and a few nuts, most vegetable proteins are "incomplete," meaning that they can build body protein only when they are combined with other vegetable sources.

If you are a vegetarian, you probably know the many ways you can build complete protein from complementary sources without consuming animal products. However, strict vegetarians may need to include cheese, eggs, or milk in addition to extra vitamin B_{12} to prepare for a healthy pregnancy.

Fruits and Vegetables—Six to Eight Servings a Day.
Fruits and vegetables are the complex carbohydrate foods containing a wide range of valuable nutrients (Bs, A, E, and C, plus minerals), along with fiber which is necessary for proper digestion. Complex carbohydrates should constitute as much as 60 percent of the total calories in your diet, which is equivalent to about four to six servings daily of vegetables (starchy and nonstarchy) and at least two servings of fresh fruit.

Fruits and vegetables can deliver optimum nutrition if they are fresh and not overcooked. Eat as many kinds of vegetables and fruits as possible, raw as well as cooked. Choose fresh before frozen, and frozen before canned. It's a good idea to peel most fresh fruits and vegetables because chemical sprays, colorants, and other contaminants are concentrated in the skin. When cooking vegetables, try steaming rather than boiling in order to retain valuable nutrients. Pure fruit and vegetable juices and dried fruit, such as raisins, dates, and figs, also fall into this group.

Grains and Cereals—Two Servings a Day.
Choose unrefined foods, such as whole grain breads and cereals, brown rice, and whole wheat pastas. Whole grains are important sources of B vitamins, fiber, iron, magnesium, and nutrients crucial to pregnancy.

Essential Fats and Oils—Two to Three Tablespoons a Day
Essential fatty acids are vital for proper development of the nervous system in the fetus, and for the regulation of a class of hormones called prostaglandins which help regulate inflammation and cellular immunity, and which stimulate contractions of the uterus. Essential fatty acids are found mainly in vegetable oils, nuts, and nut butters. Other rich sources include soy, corn, safflower, linseed, and peanut oils; avocado and wheat germ also contain substantial amounts. These oils should be cold-pressed (not processed) and kept refrigerated at all times.

Avoid hydrogenated oils, margarines, or all-purpose oils that have been heated, bleached, or otherwise altered. Fresh butter in small amounts is better than these hydrogenated fats.

Animal fats supply only tiny amounts of essential fatty acids. If you vary your diet, you will be getting plenty of saturated fat from sources such as whole milk, meat, oily fish, cheese, and egg yolk. Your total fat intake—both animal fats and vegetables oils—before and during pregnancy should not exceed 20 to 25 percent of the total calories in your diet, and most of these should come from vegetable oils.

Foods to Avoid
Now is the time to stop drinking alcohol. One or two glasses of wine a week probably aren't going to hurt you, but because part of the objective of the Pre-Pregnancy Diet is to cleanse your system, the three-month advance plan is a perfect time to detox.

In addition to alcohol, avoid processed foods and those containing artificial additives. These include processed cheeses, some meat products—such as sausages and luncheon meat—certain frozen foods, and many canned and packaged foods. Avoid white bread and other highly processed or oversweetened baked goods. Sugary foods—candies, cakes, cookies, soft drinks—offer no nutrient content. Choose instead whole grain, high-fiber breads and cereals and fruit and vegetable juices.

The contents of many packaged foods are required by law to be declared on the label, so get into the habit of reading labels before you buy things.

Try to eat as little canned food as possible and then only the foods whose nutritional content is least affected by the canning process, such as tuna, sardines, tomatoes, and pineapple. If you buy canned fruit, choose those canned in their own juice instead of in syrup. It's also best to keep to the minimum salted snacks and nuts, and to avoid margarines.

SAMPLE PRE-PREGNANCY MENUS
1,400–1,600 calories
per day

DAY 1

Breakfast

A whole orange, sliced
1 cup whole grain cereal (cooked)
with
1 tsp. maple syrup
1 oz. sunflower seeds
1 oz. raisins
1 cup low-fat milk

Lunch

2 oz. cheddar or 4 oz. cottage cheese
Large garden salad with fresh greens, alfalfa sprouts, ½ avocado
Salad dressing with 1 tbs. vegetable or olive oil

Snack

2 rice crackers with 1 tsp. natural peanut butter or
tahini (sesame butter)

Dinner

4–6 oz. veal sautéed in 2 pats of butter with scallions
Steamed asparagus
½ cup brown rice or wild rice
Steamed chard or spinach

DAY 2

Breakfast

1/2 fresh papaya or whole pear or whole banana
1 cup plain yogurt with
1 tsp. honey and 1 oz. (10–12) almonds or
pecans

Lunch

Broiled chicken (6 oz.)
Small sweet potato and 1 pat of butter
Steamed kale or beet greens
Steamed yellow squash or zucchini

Snack

1/2 fresh papaya or canteloupe

Dinner

Shrimp, crab,
scallops, oysters, or clams (6 oz.)
Steamed string beans with 1 oz. slivered almonds and 1–2 pats
butter or 1 tbs. vegetable oil
1/2 cup black beans or lentils

DAY 3

Breakfast

2 eggs, poached or scrambled
2 slices whole wheat toast with 2 pats of butter
3 dried figs or prunes
1/2 fresh grapefruit
1 cup low-fat milk

Lunch

Broiled lamb chop (lean) or pork chop (lean)
1 cup steamed carrots with parsley and 1 pat of butter

Cucumber slices, watercress, or arugula
Salad dressing with
1 tbs. vegetable or olive oil

Snack

2 tangerines
1 oz. (10–12) hazelnuts or cashews

Dinner

1 cup whole grain pasta or grain main dish: kasha, barley, millet,
or wheat taboula salad with 1 tsp. sesame seeds or
1/2 cup chick peas
1–2 cups steamed vegetables (broccoli, squash, string beans)

DAY 4

Breakfast

2 oz. smoked fish or 3 oz. poached salmon
1 cup of oatmeal, cooked, with 1 pat of butter, honey (1 tsp.),
currants, or raisins (1 oz.)

Lunch

3 oz. sliced turkey
Baked potato with 1 pat of butter and chives or parsley
Green salad with
1 tbs. vegetable or olive oil dressing

Snack

Apple or orange (whole)
1 cup low-fat milk

Dinner

4–6 oz. broiled or baked fish: fresh trout, halibut, or tuna
1/2 baked squash, acorn or butternut
1/2 cup lima beans

The basis of any healthy diet is moderation and common sense. Calorie counting or measuring food is not important unless you need to gain or lose weight before pregnancy. If you follow the guidelines of the Pre-Pregnancy Diet you should be able to establish quality nutrition and create a varied menu of foods that serves both your tastes and your pre-pregnancy needs.

HOW INTERACTIONS WORK

Nutritional scientists once assumed that if a food contained a good deal of a particular nutrient it was a good dietary source of that nutrient. Thus, if you ate foods high in iron, your body would in fact absorb and be nourished by iron. In recent years a more sophisticated understanding of how nutrients are absorbed through the intestines into the body has led to a rethinking of how food is used. We know now that vitamins and minerals interact, and certain foods may interfere with—or aid—the absorption of nutrients.

For example, vitamin C, vitamin A, and adequate protein make it possible for the body to absorb iron. The iron salts found in iron supplements destroy vitamin E, which means that other vitamins and numerous hormones become damaged. Moreover, iron supplements increase the need for pantothenic acid, vitamin C, and oxygen, all vital to the developing fetus.

And without magnesium and vitamin D the body doesn't properly use calcium. Certain high-fiber foods are known to reduce the body's ability to absorb essential minerals such as iron and calcium. We also have learned that certain raw foods contain antinutrients—absorption inhibitors—that can only be destroyed by cooking.

Knowledge of these complex interactions leads scientists to confirm what your mother has been saying all your life: the key to good health is a varied and well-balanced diet. Still, some people are particularly vulnerable to interaction problems. According to the Institute of Food Technologists, a nonprofit professional society in Chicago, people at risk include faddists, dieters, and people with diet-restricting health problems, all of whom habitually eat unbalanced diets; those on long-term medication or those who abuse alcohol or drugs; or those who self medicate with megadoses of vitamins, minerals, or micronutrients. Excessive amounts of zinc, for example, can cause a type of anemia associated with a copper deficiency. Zinc megadoses also inhibit calcium absorption if dietary calcium is already low. The underlying message that the study of nutrient interactions offers is as follows. Eat a varied diet; rotate foods (avoid relying on the same things day after day); stay away from megadoses of vitamins and minerals. Blanch or cook most of the foods and vegetables that contain antinutrients; these include: legumes, eggs, raw fish and shellfish, brussels sprouts and red cabbage, cauliflower, kale, turnips, rutabagas. Diets based on a narrow selection of foods or food combinations, though often popular and trendy, may lead to interaction problems. The wider your selection from the high-quality, high-nutrient foods outlined in the Pre-Pregnancy Diet, the better your condition going into pregnancy.

ACHIEVING NORMAL WEIGHT BEFORE PREGNANCY

Once you become pregnant it's too late to start dieting or changing your basic body weight in either direction. To avoid the problems inherent in underweight/overweight pregnancy it's important to get as close as possible to an ideal weight before you conceive. If you are very thin or extremely overweight you do not want to merely add or deduct fat, but also to enhance nutrition. Here are some things you should know.

Overweight

No matter how heavy you are when you become pregnant you should not try to seriously cut down on your eating during pregnancy. Pregnancy is not the time to get rid of pre-pregnancy fat because you risk omitting from your diet some nutrients the baby needs for normal development. Also, as you lose weight body fat is broken down into substances called ketone bodies which are passed to the fetus where they can damage its developing brain and body.

If you are a chronic dieter and perpetually overweight, the need to eat well and gain weight during pregnancy may be difficult to accept. In fact, I've known some overweight women to welcome morning sickness because they thought they could lose some weight and come out on the other side of pregnancy slimmer than when they began. The baby cannot live off your body fat. It must have a continuous supply of nutrients over the nine-month gestational period if it is to develop normally. Slightly lower weight gains appear to be all right for extremely overweight pregnant women, but overall your baby will be better off if you eat nourishing foods and gain an appropriate amount of weight.

Susan Shaw points out that being a little overweight is not thought to be harmful to pregnancy. But, says Shaw, if you have an average body frame and are thirty or more pounds overweight, then you have reached the point where you should lose weight before becoming pregnant. Use a standard table of height/weight ratio; if you are 20 percent over or under the criteria you need to do something about it.

Because it's possible to be overweight and still be malnourished, it's important to choose a gradual form of weight loss that also enhances your nutritional status. Do not go on a crash diet before pregnancy. Any extreme form of diet risks depleting essential nutrients from your body that you need for a healthy pregnancy.

The Best Weight-Loss Program Before Pregnancy

Any weight-loss program you choose before pregnancy should be protein-sparing. This means that you take in enough protein to replace the amount of protein being used by your muscles. But you don't take in enough to cause weight gain. A good protein-sparing diet is low in fat (10 percent), moderate in carbohydrates (40 percent), and relatively high in high-quality protein (50 percent). Such a program has the benefits of a low-calorie diet, without the hazards of muscle wasting. It sets the stage for fat loss while maintaining the body's blood sugar levels and energy.

Studies indicate that calorie levels as low as six to eight hundred calories a day were safely maintained on this kind of program over prolonged periods. However, a more gradual weight-loss program, between eight and twelve hundred calories a day, is better in preparation for pregnancy.

The protein can come from a variety of lean meats, fish, eggs, or cheese—or from a well-balanced protein powder made from a variety of sources. (Soy powder alone is insufficient.) Even if you include skim milk in your weight-loss diet, you will need a calcium supplement to get your calcium intake up to sufficient pre-pregnancy levels.

Carbohydrates should be balanced between whole grains and starchy vegetables (cereal, yams, potatoes) and green vegetables. Carbohydrates can also include small amounts of unrefined sugar foods such as fruits and vegetable juices. (You should dilute fruit juices.) There should be enough fiber from vegetables and whole grains in the diet to promote intestinal regularity and prevent constipation. If not, a natural fiber such as oat bran or flax seeds may be added daily.

Some vitamins and minerals may need to be supplemented—this depends on your physical condition. It is essential to combine any weight-loss program with exercise, particularly aerobic exercise.

Underweight

Can you ever be too thin? If you are thin and tend to tire quickly and are prone to frequent colds and other minor ailments, and you can't seem to add any weight, the answer is yes.

The first step you should take is to make sure you aren't suffering from any illness. Anemia, juvenile onset diabetes, an overactive thyroid, and digestive problems can all prevent nutrients from being absorbed and properly used. Depression is also frequently associated with extreme thinness, as is anorexia nervosa, a kind of self-induced starvation undertaken by some women who perceive themselves as fat no matter how thin they become. All of these conditions need to be properly diagnosed and treated by specialists before you attempt to become pregnant.

Most of the time, however, thinness is simply traced to poor eating patterns. Nutritionists say that many underweight people eat virtually nothing throughout the day and only a small meal at night. Erratic eating habits are another common cause. Sometimes people become underweight because of temporary stress or illness.

Most problems can be solved simply by boosting caloric intake. This does not mean empty calories found in soda pop, candy, or junk food, however. Forget about milk shakes and french fries and chocolate éclairs. Fried foods and sweets will quickly add weight, but in the process can wreck your nutritional balance.

If you need to gain weight, concentrate on the nutritious foods: whole nuts and seeds and nut butters, ounce for ounce, are more caloric than most foods and an excellent source of vitamin E, magnesium, and essential fatty acids. Dried fruits—raisins, apricots, prunes—are packed with vitamins A and C and are a good source of potassium and iron. Sweet potatoes have twice the number of calories as white potatoes and supply more vitamin A and minerals. Avocados are also high in calories and nutrients.

If you choose not to eat protein such as meat, fish, or eggs, a well-balanced protein powder can be taken instead. Choose a product without sugar which can be mixed in milk or fresh fruit juice. Snack throughout the day on whole grain products, fruit, and nuts.

If you are still underweight when you conceive, you should try to gain thirty to thirty-six pounds during pregnancy, but don't go overboard. Unless you were very underweight before pregnancy or are carrying twins or triplets, gaining more than forty pounds will not help you or your baby.

WHEN TO CONSULT A NUTRITIONIST

Obesity or a condition of extreme underweight may well require some outside help from a physician or qualified nutritionist. There are other conditions that also benefit from expert consultation.

If you suspect you have food allergies, it's important to go to a nutritionist and/or an allergist who is nutritionally oriented, because many allergies are actually a result of nutritional deficiencies. Before pregnancy you need to know if you have any food allergy, especially an allergy to any protein, so an optimum diet can be designed especially for you.

Another reason to consult a nutritionist before pregnancy is if you have diabetes or low blood sugar. A specialist can plan a diet for you that will compensate for this. It is well known that diabetic women have a greater risk of complications during pregnancy. But recent research suggests that women who have low blood sugar, or hypoglycemia, may have an even greater risk of complications. A combination of vitamins and minerals, including 100 mcg of chromium, can help maintain the proper level of sugar in the blood. The best food sources of chromium are liver, whole grains, and chromium-enriched brewer's yeast. If you have diabetes or any other disease you will also need to consult a specialist in that disorder before pregnancy. (See Chapter 14.)

Other problems that may be nutritionally related are: bleeding gums, unexplained water retention, bloating after meals, nail problems, chronic anemia, fatigue, hair loss, chronic skin problems, and poor digestion.

If you suffer from any of these conditions, you should consider having your nutritional status checked by a professional.

How Experts Check Nutritional Status

Nutritionists have several ways to check your nutritional status. To evaluate the possibility of a vitamin or mineral deficiency, a nutritionist will look for external signs and symptoms, paying special attention to certain areas of the body, such as muscles, eyes, mouth, hair, nails, and skin.

A nutritionist can also assess the general quality of your diet by using laboratory tests to measure the levels of vitamins and minerals in various body substances, including blood, urine, and saliva. Sophisticated testing of amino acid levels reveals how your body is using protein. Essential fatty acids can also be checked in the blood.

Although not an adequate diagnostic tool when used alone, hair analysis combined with blood and urine assays is a reliable indicator of exposure to toxic heavy metals such as lead, mercury, and cadmium. Within a less defined range hair analysis is also a fairly reliable indicator of zinc and chromium levels. All other applications of hair analysis are controversial.

AFTER YOU BECOME PREGNANT: HOW DIET AFFECTS PREGNANCY

The first study that examined the influence of a mother's diet on the health of her baby was performed in England in 1916. Researchers found that babies born to malnourished women were more frequently premature and smaller than expected for the length of gestation. More of the babies born to poorly nourished mothers died than those born to women who were well nourished.

Several later studies analyzed the effect of wartime conditions on pregnancy and drew similar conclusions. After World War II researchers at Harvard University found conclusive evidence that a woman's diet during pregnancy influenced her newborn's birth weight, length, and general health.

HOW MUCH WEIGHT CAN YOU EXPECT TO GAIN DURING PREGNANCY?

There is no one weight gain figure that's right for every woman. A breakthrough in our understanding of weight gain came in the late 1960s when Dr. Nicholson J. Eastman of Johns Hopkins University studied twelve thousand pregnancies and found that babies had a better chance of surviving if their mothers gained at least twenty pounds during pregnancy. About twenty pounds can be accounted for by growth of the fetus and its supporting tissues and fluids, and by maternal changes, such as heavier breasts, that are essential to a healthy pregnancy. An extra few pounds are recommended to provide nutritional leeway for the mother and baby. Many obstetricians today opt for even higher figures.

The American College of Obstetricians and Gynecologists recommends that women entering pregnancy near their ideal weight should gain twenty-five to thirty pounds during pregnancy. And underweight woman may have to gain as much as thirty-five pounds to ensure her baby's proper development. An overweight woman should eat nutritiously, and with the advice of her obstetrician, may plan to gain slightly less than the recommended amount.

HOW WEIGHT IS DISTRIBUTED IN PREGNANCY

The weight you gain during the first half of your pregnancy goes into building up stores of fat and protein that can be used by your baby later in the pregnancy. Some of these stores will be held over to sustain you after pregnancy and to help produce breast milk.

Rate of Gain

Ideally you should gain weight steadily throughout pregnancy, rather than in spurts. During the first three months you should gain a total of two to five pounds, and three to four pounds a month thereafter. If you've gained too much weight over the course of pregnancy, do *not* cut back toward the end. The weight increase during the last three months represents mostly growth of the baby, so a cutback in calories then could compromise the baby's development.

The way you eat and what you eat are more important than the precise amount of weight you gain. Weight gain should be gradual and consistent—and the best way to manage that is by eating a well-balanced diet.

How Much Should the Baby Weigh

A mother's diet sets up a chain reaction: diet affects the child's birth weight, and birth weight is closely related to the child's future health and development. In other words, a child born underweight has a hard time making up that disadvantage in later years. A large study funded by the National Institutes of Health found that babies weighing seven pounds six ounces or more had fewer diseases and were generally healthier than babies who weighed less. In another study in Detroit, children who had been in the highest average weight group at birth had the highest average IQ test scores; those with the lowest birth weights had significantly lower scores.

Although bigger babies tend to do better, extremely large babies do not. Babies weighing more than ten pounds at birth have a somewhat higher than average number of problems during labor and delivery. The birth of babies weighing more than ten pounds, however, is not usually related to high weight gains during pregnancy. It is most often associated with pre-pregnancy obesity, poorly controlled diabetes during pregnancy, pregnancy lasting longer than forty-two weeks, or a family history of large newborns.

How much a baby weighs in relationship to his or her gestational age (length of pregnancy) is the best indicator of health. A small-for-dates baby is more likely to have trouble than a small baby who is the right size for its gestational age. So if a six-and-a-half-pound baby is born after eight months, it is likely to experience fewer health complications than if it weighed the same after nine months.

RETURNING TO YOUR NORMAL WEIGHT

You will not lose all the weight you gained immediately after delivery. Some of that weight will be stored as fat to aid you in breast-feeding. Even if you don't plan to breast-feed, the fat you require for milk production will be deposited automatically by your body. Do not cut back on weight gain because you don't expect to breast-feed. Your body will still deposit the fat you require for milk production, if necessary taking away essential nutrients from the fetus.

During the first week after delivery you can expect to lose about fifteen pounds. That includes the baby, the placenta, and extra fluids. From then on, if you're nursing the baby, you can expect to lose about a half pound a week. On average, breast-feeding mothers are naturally back to their normal weight by six weeks after delivery. Bottle-feeding mothers tend to lose weight more slowly. If you've trained yourself to eat properly, weight loss will be automatic and without stress.

If you were overweight before pregnancy (or if you gain more than forty pounds during pregnancy), you'll be overweight after delivery. If you don't breast-feed, you'll need to make an extra effort to exercise more and eat less, but don't try to lose more than about half a pound to one pound a week. All new mothers need to conserve energy, so avoid crash weight-loss programs.

Nutrition plays a vital part in our ability to function at the highest possible level, both emotionally and physically. And when preparing for pregnancy, you want all the advantages of a proper diet not only for yourself, but for your child.

But diet is not the only important element for healthy life and motherhood. Exercise and physical fitness provide another vital link in preparing the body for pregnancy.

CHAPTER 11

GETTING IN SHAPE FOR PREGNANCY

PREGNANCY IS HARD WORK; labor and delivery are even harder, and women who are physically fit seem to be able to stand the stress and strain better than women who are out of shape. Every woman should prepare for pregnancy by getting physically fit. Fitness first —pregnancy second. It's safer to continue exercising during pregnancy if your body is already in shape.

Women who wait to start an exercise program after they become pregnant can't really prepare themselves properly because of the limitations imposed by pregnancy. For example, it's not easy to strengthen back muscles while you are pregnant. Another reason to get in shape early is that if you suffer from nausea and fatigue in the early months of your pregnancy you will find it difficult to exercise.

Pregnancy is like an athletic event: the longer and more sensibly you train for it, the better your endurance and stamina will be.

The goal of a pre-pregnancy exercise program is to maintain good health throughout pregnancy and afterward, and to avoid some of the aches and pains of pregnancy, including backache, loss of urinary control, hemorrhoids, and discomfort during intercourse.

Until recently there has been no direct scientific proof that women who exercise have an easier labor and delivery, only the observations of physically fit mothers themselves and some health care professionals who work with pregnant women. However, in July of 1985 two British doctors reported that women who exercise regularly are less likely to require surgical episiotomy during delivery. Obstetricians perform episiotomies to prevent tearing and damage to the perineal muscles. The researchers found that when it came to avoiding muscle damage and promoting healing, exercise was more helpful than surgical intervention.

Exercise also offers some additional benefits. A regular exercise program will stimulate your body's own repair systems. It improves circulation, tones your cardiovascular system, and tightens flabby muscles. Joints stay supple and posture improves. Regular exercise might also help to reduce emotional stress and alleviate anxiety and depression.

In addition to a general exercise program, special training exercises described in the Pre-Pregnancy Shape-Up program can be performed to strengthen the areas of the body that carry the most stress during pregnancy. After you become pregnant you can continue to perform these exercises as maintenance to stay in shape.

GENERAL EXERCISES

If you don't already exercise, the best time to begin a program is at least three months before you plan to conceive. Try to set aside about ten minutes each day for some form of exercise; if daily sessions are impractical, aim for fifteen minutes three times a week. Short, regular workouts are better for you than an hour once a week.

What kinds of exercises are best? Many different kinds of exercises can be used to increase general fitness, but if you are starting a program in preparation for pregnancy it's a good idea to choose exercises that can be continued in some form throughout pregnancy. Exercise during pregnancy is now widely recommended by most health experts. Tennis, jogging in moderation, golf, and bowling (as long as excessive twisting and bending are avoided) are also safe, as long as you become active in these sports before pregnancy. The American College of Obstetricians and Gynecologists has recently suggested that the safest and most beneficial exercises for pregnant and newly delivered mothers are brisk walking, swimming, and stationary cycling.

Marathon running, horseback riding, and sports with the potential for serious injuries (basketball, field hockey, and gymnastics) are too risky for pregnancy. Water skiing and surfing should definitely be avoided because a fall during pregnancy could result in water being forced into the vagina or rectum, leading to a variety of complications.

To get into shape for pregnancy, choose a moderately strenuous form of exercise. You may prefer a body-toning workout. If you decide on an aerobic or other exercise class, choose a program run by an experienced professional.

Whatever form of exercise you choose, take care not to go to extremes. Sustained heavy exercise, particularly running and jogging, can prevent regular ovulation, causing infertility. If you have had irregular periods or previously miscarried, check with your doctor about how much exercise is too much before deciding on an exercise program.

Start your exercise program gently. Before you embark on any change in your normal daily routine, it is always wise to consult your physician first, especially if you do not usually exercise or if you have any chronic medical condition such as asthma, hypertension, or arthritis.

SPECIFIC MUSCLES NEED SPECIFIC EXERCISES

During pregnancy hormonal changes, plus the weight of the growing fetus, cause muscles and ligaments to soften and stretch. If your muscles are well toned before you become pregnant, they will provide all the support your body needs to accommodate these changes.

Certain areas of your body—specifically the pelvic floor muscles, the abdomen, and the back—are placed under maximum stress during pregnancy. These are the areas that need the most attention. As your abdomen stretches and the baby's weight increases, the natural curve in your spine deepens, and your center of gravity is thrust slightly forward. Without strong muscular support, the pelvis will also tilt forward, setting up a misalignment that leads to the backache so common in pregnancy. Strong abdominal and back muscles that help you maintain good posture should be high on your list of exercise goals. The muscles of the pelvic floor, which help support the weight of the fetus, also need to be well toned for the time when you'll need them most—during delivery.

Exercising these muscle groups are important for all women preparing for pregnancy, especially those who are over age thirty.

Pelvic Floor Muscles
Just as everything else softens and loosens as pregnancy progresses, so do the muscles in the pelvic floor. These muscles have to carry substantial additional weight during pregnancy, and they also must be able to stretch to the maximum while the baby is being born. The improved blood circulation that comes with exercise increases their elasticity, helping the muscles stretch over the baby's head with minimal strain. If you exercise these muscles well before pregnancy, the pelvic floor will support the weight of the baby better during pregnancy and function smoothly during labor and childbirth. Well-exercised muscles will also restore themselves much sooner than those that have been neglected.

Abdominal Muscles
Stomach or abdominal muscles are often the weakest group of muscles in our bodies, and their weakness is the most common cause of backache. The same abdominal muscles that support the pelvis also support the delicate column of the spine.

Because they bear the whole torso in an upright position the abdominal muscles must be strong and firm. The stronger these muscles are, the more erect is your stance, and the easier it will be for you to carry added weight in front.

During pregnancy, as your abdominal muscles become elongated and stretch to accommodate an expanding uterus, they will become vulnerable to strain. Because of this vulnerability it is difficult to exercise and strengthen these muscles after you become pregnant.

The Back Muscles
As pregnancy progresses, your center of gravity will shift forward. Most pregnant women try to compensate for the shift by leaning farther back on their heels. This thrusts the pelvis forward, stretching the abdominal muscles even more and increasing the strain on the spine.

Strong back muscles will help keep your pelvis balanced, and the rest of your body will automatically fall into alignment. When you stand, sit, and walk with proper posture, you will be able to better carry the baby and yourself.

THE PRE-PREGNANCY SHAPE-UP

The following series of pelvic, abdominal, and back exercises has been designed especially for *The Pre-Pregnancy Planner* by Deirdre Pachón, founder of Synergetics, the Exercise Phenomenon, in New York City. If these exercises seem odd to you, says Ms. Pachón, who specializes in developing exercise programs to meet individual needs, you will understand them better after you become pregnant. When you feel your balance and center of gravity shift, you will be glad that your back is strong and your posture erect. You will also be able to adapt these same exercises at a lower level of exertion to use during pregnancy.

The following six exercises are designed to be performed in sequence, three times per week, in conjunction with your usual activity or other forms of exercise. Deep rhythmic breathing as you carry out this sequence of exercises will ensure that your entire system will become oxygenated.

THE PELVIS

#1   This exercise is designed for increasing mobility of the pelvis and lower back, strengthening the pelvic floor, and as a warm-up for the exercises that follow.

Starting Position: Begin on all fours, knees hip-width apart, your weight distributed evenly over your knees and hands.

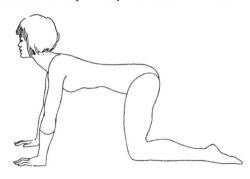

a. Inhale, then exhale as you round your back and tuck your pelvis under.

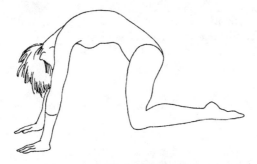

b. Circle your hips right four times, then left four times.

c. Inhale, then exhale as you round your back and pull your abdominals in and up. Hold this position. Now tighten the muscles of your buttocks, rectum, vagina, and bladder. Feel yourself contracting these muscles from within. Tighten and release eight times.

Repeat in sequence for three sets.

#2 This exercise is designed to strengthen the pelvic floor and align the lumbar spine, and it is to be used as a preparation for the abdominal exercises that follow.

Starting Position: Lie on your back, feet hip-width apart on the floor, your fingers interlaced behind your head, with your elbows resting on floor.

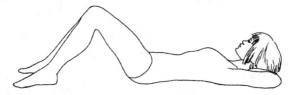

a. Inhale, then exhale as you curl your tailbone up slightly while pressing the back of your waist onto the floor. Pull your abdominals in and up so that your abdomen feels hollow.

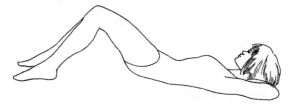

b. Tighten the muscles of your rectum, vagina, and bladder. Hold for eight seconds, then release. (Note: try to relax your buttock muscles while contracting from within.)

THE ABDOMEN

#3 and #4 The following two exercises are designed to strengthen the abdominals while releasing and building a strong support for your back.

Starting Position: Hold exercise 2 in the contracted position, supporting your head off the floor with your hands.

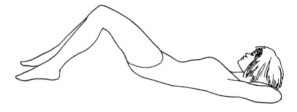

a. Inhale and exhale as you make little lifts (exhale while lifting), bringing your elbows closer to your knees. Repeat eight times.

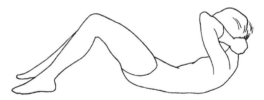

b. Inhale and exhale, bringing your right knee toward your chest and your left elbow toward your right knee. Exhale with each touch. Touch-release eight times.

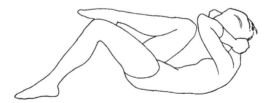

c. Rest your head on the floor. Bring your knees toward your chest. Now lift, then lower, your hips eight times. Think of tighten -

ing your abdominals while bringing your pubic bone toward your navel. (Note: try not to press your knees tightly against your chest.)

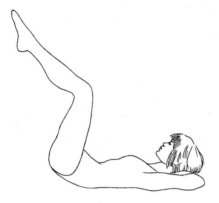

Repeat in sequence for three sets.

Starting Position: Lie on your back, knees to your chest, hands holding your knees, your elbows lifted up and out.

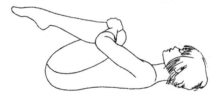

a. Pull your knees away from your chest, lift your upper back off the floor, keep your chin to your chest. Once you are up as high as you can go, inhale, then exhale, pulling your abdominals in and up, letting go of your knees, reaching out past your feet which are trying to stay up. Stay lifted for eight seconds.

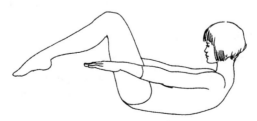

b. Inhale, and slowly fold your knees back to your chest, resting your head and back on floor.

Repeat in sequence for three sets.

THE BACK

#5 and #6 The following two exercises will give you a strong and powerful back. Don't be discouraged if your movement doesn't seem to be big. Stop if you feel pain. Build up slowly. (Note: these back exercises should not be performed if you are pregnant.)

Starting Position: Lie face down with your arms crossed under your forehead, your legs straight and together.

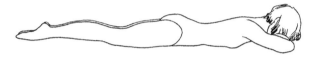

a. Inhale and exhale, pulling your abdominals in and up. Tighten your buttocks and lift both legs off the floor. Hold for eight seconds, then release.

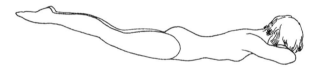

b. Keeping your buttocks tight and abdominals pulled in and up, inhale and exhale as you lift your right leg from the hip, keeping it stiff and straight. Hold it up for eight seconds. (Note: keep your hip bones on the floor.) Repeat with your other leg.

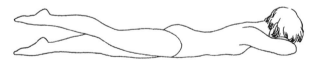

c. Optional: Interlace your fingers behind your head. Keeping your abdominals pulled in and up, inhale and lift your head and elbows (and chest, if you can) off the floor. Keep your neck straight. Don't look up. Repeat eight times.

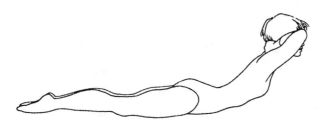

d. To release back: roll onto your back, and hug your knees to your chest. Breathe at a natural pace while holding this position for eight seconds.

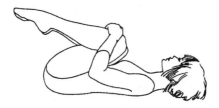

Starting Position: Sit up straight with your back against a wall. Place the soles of your feet together. Interlace your fingers behind your head, with your elbows open wide. Your feet should be a little out in front so it's comfortable to sit up straight.

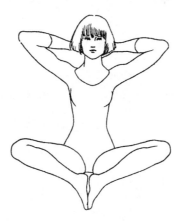

a. Inhale and exhale as you lean forward, rounding your back, bringing your elbows toward your ankles.

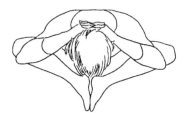

b. Inhale and exhale as you slowly come up, touching your waist, then ribs, shoulders, head, and elbows last, to the wall. Repeat four times.

c. With your back now straight, inhale. Exhale as you bring your right elbow toward your left leg. Come up. (Note: keep your buttocks on the floor when you go over.) Do the other side. Repeat four times.

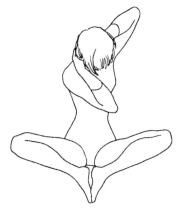

d. With your back straight and your elbows back, inhale. Exhale, then bring your right elbow toward your right hip. Bend sideways in the waist. Slowly come up. Do the other side. Repeat four times.

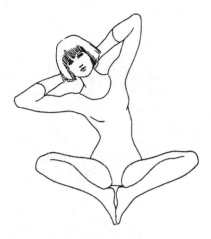

Repeat in sequence for three sets.

This section of *The Pre-Pregnancy Planner* has covered the major health and fitness components facing prospective parents today. For a quick review—and some additional tips on planning a three-month program—the Pre-Pregnancy Checklist follows. If you can assure yourself that you have covered all the points in the checklist, you know that you are ready for pregnancy.

CHAPTER 12

THE PRE-PREGNANCY CHECKLIST

As we've discussed, achieving health and fitness for pregnancy may mean breaking bad habits (smoking and junk food) and creating new ones (exercise and good nutrition). Making these changes can be stressful, and the early stages of pregnancy aren't the best time to be adding stress to your life. If your lifestyle needs a major overhaul, you're better off starting several months before conception.

A THREE-MONTH PLAN

The best plan allows at least three months to eliminate dangers and build in protections. In that time you should be able to make whatever changes seem necessary to ensure a healthy pregnancy. Changes might include switching to a safer contraceptive, adjusting diet and exercise, eliminating drugs and alcohol, and stopping smoking. If you are a heavy smoker, you will probably want to allow more than three months to break the habit.

You can analyze your present reproductive status and discover what changes you need to make by going through the Pre-Pregnancy Checklist.

The Pre-Pregnancy Checklist includes a medical checkup with your gynecologist or family physician, a visit to the dentist, and an analysis of your diet and lifestyle.

A MEDICAL CHECKUP

There are many reasons for a medical checkup before you become pregnant. First, you want to make sure that your reproductive organs are functioning properly, so that when you do choose to become pregnant you will be able to conceive. When you make your appointment, be sure to tell your physician that you are thinking about becoming pregnant and want a complete report on your reproductive status.

A pre-pregnancy medical checkup is similar to a prenatal checkup. The difference is that in this case you are not yet pregnant. The visit begins with your family medical history. Your physician should then take your blood pressure and give you a general physical examination, including an internal vaginal and pelvic exam, urinalysis, blood tests, and breast examination.

Medical History
You will be asked if you've ever had a serious illness, including kidney disease, diabetes, rubella, high blood pressure, or pelvic inflammatory disease. Your doctor will want to know if you have had any recent inoculations or if you take any medications.

A note will be made if there are any twins in your family or any history of birth defects or other serious illnesses. If you can trace an unusual incidence of a disease or birth defects in your family, you will probably want to consult a genetic counselor before becoming pregnant to assess the chances of passing along the disorder.

If you have encountered any complications in a previous pregnancy your physician will want to know about them. Miscarriage, premature birth, and preeclampsia are just a few of the conditions that may have bearing on the outcome of your next pregnancy.

Your physician will also want a description of your menstrual pattern. Menstrual problems suggest a number of possibilities that may need investigating: endometriosis, erratic ovulation, unbalanced hormonal cycles, and premature menopause are a few. If any of these problems do exist, you will want to have them treated before you try to become pregnant.

Height and Weight
On this first visit your height might be measured, which will give the physician a rough idea of whether you are ready to start pregnancy at about the right weight for your height. The measuring process will also show if you have any posture or other physical abnormalities that might affect your pelvis.

Your weight before you conceive is as important as your weight gain during pregnancy. If you have a significant weight problem in either direction, you should consult a nutritionist. It's important to add, or lose, weight *before* you become pregnant. (See Chapter 10.)

Pelvic Exam

The internal exam will detect any structural abnormalities of the pelvis, vagina, and cervix that might affect the pregnancy. During the exam the physician can take cervical swabs for a Pap smear, and to test for gonorrhea and other venereal infections.

Checks for Venereal Disease

Many potentially dangerous venereal diseases are silent. Gonorrhea is easily identified, usually by a slide test in the physician's office. However, the insidious chlamydia infection is much harder to discover. New tests are now available which can uncover a completely invisible chlamydia infection. Ask your doctor about their availability. (See Chapter 9.)

Urine Tests

Your urine specimen can be analyzed for the presence of protein, which may indicate kidney disease; glucose, which would indicate diabetes; ketones, which may indicate that you're not eating enough; pus or blood, which could be an indication of kidney infection.

Blood Tests

A blood sample is analyzed to identify your blood group, in case you need an emergency transfusion, and to test for venereal disease, anemia, and the rhesus factor. If you are Rh-negative and your partner is Rh-positive, you may potentially have a high-risk pregnancy. (See Chapter 14.)

If you are black or Hispanic, your blood can be tested for sickle-cell disease and sickle-cell trait. If both partners carry the sickle-cell trait, there is an increased risk of the baby having sickle-cell disease, a severe form of anemia. (See Chapter 13.)

If you or your partner is of southern Mediterranean ancestry, your blood may be tested for thalassemia, another hereditary blood disease that can cause severe anemia in the baby. Or if you are of

Eastern European Jewish descent, a screening test for a metabolic disorder called Tay-Sachs disease should be considered.

Your blood may also be tested for toxoplasmosis, an infection that can severely affect fetal development.

It will be tested as well for rubella antibodies. If the blood test shows that you are not immune, you can be vaccinated, as long as you are not yet pregnant.

Rubella Vaccinations

Although a relatively trivial illness, rubella can have grave consequences for an unborn baby. If a pregnant woman catches it during the first three months of pregnancy, there is a 20 to 30 percent risk that the baby's eyes, ears, brain, or heart may be damaged.

Later in pregnancy, the risk to the baby is much less, with damage usually restricted to hearing difficulties. The virus may also cause miscarriage, a low birth-weight baby, or even a stillbirth.

Even if you think you have had rubella, commonly known as German measles, or were vaccinated against it, ask your doctor to check that you are still immune. Rubella is a mild, highly infectious illness that lasts for only a few days. It often resembles other viruses —exhibiting slight rash and fever—and may have been wrongly diagnosed or your vaccination may not have taken.

If your doctor finds that you are not immune to rubella you can be vaccinated *before* you become pregnant. After you conceive you cannot be vaccinated because the live vaccine might harm the unborn child. However, as long as you do not contract German measles during pregnancy the baby will be all right. Other vaccines may be given later in pregnancy but are usually best avoided. If you are planning a trip abroad, make sure your inoculations are up to date before you try to conceive.

If you are vaccinated, it's important that you do not become pregnant for at least three months.

A DENTAL CHECKUP

No one wants to undertake extensive dental work while pregnant. There is the potential danger from X rays, drug therapy, or painkillers, as well as the stress of drilling. At the same time, you don't want to let serious dental problems go for an extended time, say, nine months, while you're waiting to have a baby. According to Dr. Malvin Braverman, former Chief of Dentistry at Montefiore Hospital's Martin Luther King Center in New York City, the answer is a pre-pregnancy dental checkup. "An evaluation of your mouth, including X rays, will tell you if you need work. If so, you can get it cleared up in advance of pregnancy. The checkup can also make sure your gums are in good shape."

It's only a myth that a baby drains the calcium from your teeth. Although the growing fetus needs calcium for its own development, it will not draw it from its mother's teeth because the calcium in teeth, unlike that in bones, is tightly bound.

The dental problems some women encounter during pregnancy are usually related to gum ailments. As a result of pregnancy hormones in the blood a pregnant woman's gums become softer and more vascular, which makes them more vulnerable to inflammation and disease.

While major dental work should be avoided when you are pregnant, good dental hygiene is a must. Dr. Braverman, who is now in private practice in New York, recommends that after a woman becomes pregnant she increase the length of time she brushes her teeth each day and schedule regular appointments with a dental hygienist for cleaning.

For good hygiene maintenance Braverman suggests brushing with a mixture of baking soda and a small amount of peroxide blended into a paste. If you have a Water Pik, add two tablespoons of peroxide to the water tank and rinse your mouth before and after brushing. This hygiene plan can be used once a week if your gums are normal, and once a day if you are experiencing gum problems.

Your gums may swell and even bleed when you are pregnant, but if you maintain good hygiene they will not become infected and cause more serious problems. After childbirth, when your regular hormonal balance resumes, your teeth and gums should be in good condition.

DIET AND LIFESTYLE

Ideally before conception you and your partner should assess your lifestyle and make any necessary changes. The effect of this preparation will increase your chances of giving birth to a healthy baby.

You will also be fitter during pregnancy and less likely to suffer from postnatal depression or inability to breast-feed. After the baby is weaned, you will be in good shape mentally and physically.

Your physician or a nutritionist can help you assess your lifestyle to pinpoint changes that might benefit you and your baby. Here are some of the things you should consider.

Diet and Exercise

Good nutrition and physical fitness are the cornerstones of a healthy pregnancy. Before you become pregnant you should get in the habit of eating a well-balanced diet. (See Chapter 10.) In conjunction, specific muscle groups under most stress during pregnancy benefit from a planned exercise program. (See Chapter 11.)

Smoking and Alcohol

The same substances hazardous during pregnancy are also best avoided while trying to conceive. This is because the embryo is at its most vulnerable in the early weeks of development, even before you know you are pregnant.

Heavy drinking has been associated with miscarriage, low birth-weight babies, and in extreme cases, certain handicaps. Smoking may increase the risk of early miscarriage and fetal handicaps.

Certain drugs are known to endanger the fetus during pregnancy. Even drugs taken near the time of conception can be hazardous, since it is in the first few weeks of life that a baby's vital organs are forming.

Before you stop contraception, both partners should stop smoking and taking all drugs, including aspirin. The safe level of alcohol consumption during pregnancy has not been established. Moderation is the key for both partners. Reduce drinking to one or two drinks a week, or to be on the safe side, eliminate alcohol completely. (See Chapter 7.)

If you are taking prescribed drugs for a specific medical condition, do not stop or alter the regimen without consulting your physician. (See Chapter 14.)

Toxins and Pollutants

If either of you works with toxic materials, or if you live or work in a polluted atmosphere, you may need some advice from an obstetrician about possible hazards to your proposed pregnancy. (See Chapter 8.)

Contraceptives

If you have used the pill or have had problems with an IUD, it's a good idea to switch to a barrier method of contraception (condom or diaphragm) for at least three months, until you are ready to conceive. (See Chapter 9.)

Must Your Cat Go?

Toxoplasmosis, a parasitic infection which may cause spontaneous abortion, stillbirth, and fetal abnormalities, periodically gains attention because it is often transmitted by household cats—via the litter box. But the organism can be found too in the feces of infected rodents, cattle, and other animals. It can also be contracted by eating raw or undercooked meat.

Does this mean that before becoming pregnant you should put your cat up for adoption? Probably not. Before a cat can pass the disease on to you it must be infected, and cats who live indoors usually remain disease-free. If your cat is a roamer, however, you can avoid infection by keeping it off tabletops and work surfaces; washing your hands carefully before preparing food or eating; and getting someone else to empty the cat's litter box. Because neighborhood cats may stray into your backyard and use it for a cat box, it's a good idea to wear gloves when gardening.

If you have a cat, you can ask your doctor to check for toxoplasmosis in your pre-pregnancy blood test.

Surname Snags

You've agreed: he keeps his name, and you keep yours. But whose name will your jointly conceived baby carry? Even if the two of you can decide, the hospital in which you give birth may argue the point. One couple wanted to hyphenate their last names to create a new surname for the child, but the hospital refused until a lawyer gave them a legal opinion.

If you do not agree, something that occasionally comes up when couples separate or divorce before the baby is born, things can be even stickier. Only in New Hampshire and Pennsylvania do state statutes treat a child's surname as a decision of the custodial parent.

In some hospitals, before a father's name can be included on the birth certificate, couples with different last names will be asked for a marriage license or a notarized statement from the father acknowledging paternity.

The best idea is to decide ahead of time what surname you will use for your child, and clear the way by checking with your hospital and physician. You don't want the question to come up after you've delivered and you are signing the birth certificate.

Every woman and man contemplating parenthood know they are making a big decision. Long before conception you should think about the many ways your life will change. How well the pregnancy goes and how healthy the baby is depend a lot on the mother's nutrition and well-being, beginning almost the moment you decide you may want to have a child. The things you do for yourself now —before conception—can influence your baby's future.

The Pre-Pregnancy Checklist offers a condensed view of what couples can do before conception to contribute to the future wellbeing of their offspring. It applies to all couples contemplating pregnancy. However, there are certain groups of men and women who have special problems entering pregnancy. The following section of *The Pre-Pregnancy Planner* is devoted to those couples who must sort out some very special issues when they make the choice to become parents. These include couples at risk for birth defects, women who have preexisting diseases or a history of miscarriage, women over age thirty-five, and couples who are infertile.

PART THREE

SPECIAL PRE-PREGNANCY CONSIDERATIONS

CHAPTER 13

GENETIC COUNSELING
BEFORE PREGNANCY

GENETIC RESEARCH into DNA has made tremendous advances in recent years, yet modern genetics is like an infant who has struggled to its feet for the first time: it's a magificent accomplishment, but it's still a long way from walking. Even with so much more to learn, many couples who a few years ago would have been afraid to have a baby because a first child or a relative had a crippling disorder can now have pre-pregnancy counseling that helps them to have healthy children. After pregnancy begins, other new tests can be performed on the fetus to determine how the child is developing.

Birth defects affect approximately two hundred and fifty thousand American babies every year, or about 5 percent of all live-born infants, which means that 95 percent of all babies are perfectly healthy. Even if you have had a previously affected child, the chances that your next pregnancy will be normal are extremely good.

There is a misconception that if everyone had genetic screening before pregnancy birth defects would be eliminated. In fact, genetic screening cannot predict the majority of birth defects. Most congenital abnormalities strike without warning and without apparent cause. No couple, no matter how perfect their genes seem to be, is immune to a spontaneous genetic mishap. All of us carry some defective genes, although most of the time they never show up in our offspring. Environmental events also may conspire to affect the fetus during the crucial weeks immediately following conception.

Geneticists argue convincingly that everyone could benefit to some degree from screening, but for the time being screening is too lengthy and complex to be made generally available.

Having made the point, there are certain instances in which genetic counseling is invaluable. Certain people are known to be at greater risk for passing on genetic defects than are the rest of the population. It is these high-risk groups that are helped by genetic screening.

Genetic screening is recommended for couples with these well-recognized risk factors:

You previously gave birth to a child with birth defects.

Either of you has relatives born with birth defects or relatives who were known to be infertile.

You have suffered more than three early miscarriages—about 7 percent of couples who sustain multiple miscarriages have a chromosome problem.

You have had even one miscarriage in which the fetus was malformed.

You belong to an ethnic or racial group at high risk for a specific genetic disease (blacks, Hispanics, Eastern European Jews, and people from southern Mediterranean countries).

One or both of you have been exposed to high doses of radiation, drugs, or other environmental agents that could result in congenital abnormalities.

You are over age thirty-five.

If you or your partner fall into any high-risk category you could both benefit from genetic screening before you become pregnant. Single men and women in these categories who feel that having children is essential to their future happiness should consider screening even before marriage. In any case, the sooner you know the odds, the more time you will have to examine your options and make choices.

Not all birth defects are severe; many are mild mental or physical handicaps. But some are cruel and devastating disorders that lead to much suffering and early death of the child. While only a small percentage of babies suffer such serious disorders, any prospective parent who falls into one of the high-risk categories will want to know the extent of the risk.

Genetic screening tells you the *odds* of your having a child with a genetic disease, based on physical evidence. Many couples who believe they are at risk are relieved to discover through genetic screening that the risk is actually much less than they expected. Even when you have one child with a genetically transmitted defect, it doesn't mean that another child born to you will have the same problems. The risk may be high, moderate, or slim.

Sometimes a defect in a first child or in a relative may not have been inherited at all. Rubella during pregnancy is one example of an outside environmental factor that can cause severe birth defects in the developing fetus but cannot be passed on to subsequent pregnancies.

Few birth defects have a single genetic cause. Most are believed to result from the interaction of several genes, possibly in combination with environmental influences. As a result, birth defects usually occur irregularly and unpredictably.

Only a handful of laboratories are capable of doing new tests that examine genes for defects. Chromosomes, although seldom the cause of birth defects, are more easily examined. Chromosome analysis of a couple is recommended when a woman consistently aborts, or if an aborted fetus shows an abnormal chromosome pattern.

COUNSELING

Genetic counseling not only explains the risks of having a child with a certain disorder and what that disorder means. It also offers the couple alternatives for dealing with the risk.

Counseling is available from medical specialists and through such organizations as the March of Dimes. A genetic counselor is either a physician with advanced training in genetics or a nonmedical person who holds a degree in genetic counseling.

You should go to a genetic counselor prepared with as many medical records as you can gather. When you phone for an appointment, the counselor will describe the kind of background information he or she is looking for. Try to discover the medical history of your parents, brothers and sisters, grandparents, and aunts and uncles. The counselor will ask numerous questions and draw up a detailed medical genealogy chart, called a pedigree, possibly going back two or more generations.

Depending on the indicators, the counselor may request blood tests or a chromosome count for one or both of you. The counselor evaluates all of the accumulated information and calculates the probable risks of passing on a genetic defect. He or she also talks to you about options, which may include artificial insemination with donor sperm or adoption.

Sometimes chromosomal testing shows that you are biologically incapable of conception; this knowledge frees you to pursue adoption, without the years of struggle with fertility testing and treatment.

Depending on the level of risk, some couples choose for the woman to become pregnant, or continue an existing pregnancy, hoping the child won't be seriously handicapped. The risk is somewhat muted by new prenatal tests which allow the fetus to be tested in utero in the early months of pregnancy. If the developing fetus proves to be severely handicapped the parents then have the option of abortion. Specialists advise that such testing of the fetus cannot reveal the majority of birth defects, nor will it usually reveal the severity of the handicap.

Abortion is a profoundly emotional and disturbing event. It's important that before a high-risk couple creates a fetus that they discuss their options and their feelings fully *before* pregnancy and resolve the question of what to do if the fetus proves defective. Even with this preparation, the emotional climate may be so intense that should prenatal testing prove that the child is handicapped one or both partners may be unable to cope with their earlier decision.

Many couples are willing to accept the burdens of a handicapped child but cannot bear the thought of the child suffering. If they cannot accept abortion, some high-risk couples decide to avoid pregnancy and seek adoption.

Family Medical Records
Family medical records are an essential part of genetic counseling. As scientists learn more about genetic and environmental factors, they are better able to see how inherited traits interact with outside influences such as infections, medications, X rays, and drugs before and after birth.

Such a record is valuable throughout a person's life. An ideal time to start keeping a family medical history is before a family is planned, or even before marriage. Faithfully kept, it can be a useful diagnostic tool in all future medical consultations for you and your children.

HOW GENETIC DISORDERS ARE PASSED ON

Normal development of every human being depends on genetic information transmitted by both parents at the moment of conception. Every cell in the body contains a nucleus that holds a blueprint for the construction of the whole human being. Each particular cell, however, uses only the fraction of the total blueprint. Thus, some cells specialize in nerves, others in muscles, others in skin or other organs.

The total blueprint is composed of twenty-three pairs of sausage-shaped structures called chromosomes—one of each pair donated by the mother, the other by the father. The sperm and egg each possess half of a set; when they unite at conception, a complete twenty-three-pair set is reconstituted.

Within each chromosome are literally thousands of genes. The color of your eyes and the shape of your ears, as well as the indispensable components of your heart and nervous system are controlled by the action of one or more pairs of genes.

Among the vast quantity of genes, a few are likely to be abnormal; fortunately, a normal gene of one parent usually overshadows a faulty gene donated by the other parent. Despite the presence of the potentially damaging gene in the child, no genetic disease results. Most genetic diseases occur only if both parents transmit the same faulty gene, which occurs rarely.

When genetic elements conspire and a child is born with a defect, the odds that a future brother or sister will have the same problem depend on how many genes are responsible. For example, cleft lip is caused by the interaction of many genes, often combined with environmental factors. There is at least a 95 percent chance *against* the same multiple genes combining to affect a subsequent child. This is also true for structural defects of the central nervous system, such as open spine (spina bifida).

On the other hand, when a disease is caused by only two defective genes, one from each parent, as is the case with the life-threatening sickle-cell anemia, the risk for each child rises dramatically: 25 percent, or one chance in four for each pregnancy.

And when the disease is caused by a single dominant gene donated by one parent, each child has a 50 percent chance of inheriting the disorder.

Genetic disorders fall into three categories: (1) an abnormality in the chromosomes, (2) a single-gene defect, and (3) a combination of multiple-gene defects, often combined with environmental factors.

CHROMOSOMES

Chromosomal abnormalities are rarely inherited. Thus, when a birth defect is caused by a flawed chromosome, it is usually a onetime-only occurrence—something that goes wrong spontaneously at the moment of conception. A chromosome abnormality can occur because there is an extra or a missing chromosome or damage to an existing chromosome.

Most chromosomal errors have serious medical consequences and many result in miscarriage. This is nature's way of handling severely defective embryos. The classic example of a chromosomal birth defect is Down's syndrome, in which the ovum drags an extra chromosome along with it before it is fertilized.

Down's Syndrome

Down's syndrome, the most common chromosomal abnormality, is almost always a spontaneous chromosomal accident. Each cell in the body contains a fixed number of chromosomes—twenty-three pairs, or a total of forty-six. The only exceptions are reproductive cells—sperm and ova—which must reduce themselves to twenty-three single-stranded chromosomes before fertilization. In Down's syndrome chromosome number twenty-one doesn't separate properly during cell division, and the egg carries a double-stranded chromosome. When the ovum is fertilized, it gains another chromosome number twenty-one from the sperm. The result is a new cell fusion in which the twenty-first chromosome has three strands of genetic coding instead of two. Every new cell that develops from the original conception duplicates the flawed chromosome, affecting the development of numerous body structures.

A Down's syndrome baby usually has a flat face with slanting eyes, a snub nose, and often a protruding tongue. The baby's muscles lack tone and he or she may have defects of the heart, eyes, and ears. Down's syndrome causes mental retardation because the brain, as well as other body structures, is poorly developed. Down's syndrome is incurable, but the degree of retardation varies from mild to severe. There is only a small chance that Down's syndrome will recur in the same family. However, the chromosome defect occasionally is inherited, and if there is a history of Down's syndrome in your family it is wise to have genetic screening. For some reason, mothers at highest risk for recurrence seem to be those who had a Down's syndrome child when they were younger than twenty-nine. Here the chance of having another child with Down's syndrome is about 1 percent.

Although a Down's syndrome baby can be born to a mother of any age, older women are known to have a greater risk. The overall incidence is about one in six hundred and fifty live births, but the incidence rises consistently for older women, and reaches one in fifty for mothers over the age of forty. New data show that the risk increases gradually and steadily as a woman grows older, rather than rising sharply at about age thirty-five, as was previously thought.

An increased risk is also suspected when the father is over the age of forty-one, but additional studies have yet to confirm that father's age is a significant factor. A genetics counselor will advise older couples of the odds of conceiving a Down's syndrome child.

Many couples at risk for Down's syndrome decide to go ahead and have a child; they either commit themselves to accepting the outcome, or they rely on new prenatal testing—amniocentesis or chorionic villi biopsy—which can detect problems in the fetus long before birth.

SINGLE-GENE DEFECTS

Single-gene defects, which affect approximately 1 percent of newborns, can be traced to isolated genes in one or both parents. These are the defects that can be most accurately predicted by genetic screening. They fall into three categories: dominant- , recessive- , and sex-linked-gene defects.

Dominant Genes

When a child is born with a dominant-gene defect, perhaps missing a little finger, one of its parents usually has a similar defect. If one parent has a dominant gene for a disease, there is a 50 percent risk that the parent will pass the gene to each child, and the child will manifest the defect. There is an equal likelihood that the child will not receive the abnormal gene.

Dominant diseases may look different in different members of a family. So if one of your parents is known to be affected, the genetic counselor will want you to receive a careful physical examination to make sure you aren't displaying some minor form of the disorder. If you are free of the defect, you will not transmit the disease.

Currently well over a thousand dominant disorders have been catalogued. They include: achondroplasia, a form of dwarfism; Huntington's disease, the progressive degeneration of the nervous system; polydactyly, extra fingers or toes; chronic simple glaucoma; and hypercholesterolemia, or high blood cholesterol levels, with a propensity to heart disease.

Recessive Genes

The second group of severe genetic diseases in which a genetics counselor can predict the risk are known as recessive-inheritance diseases. Many of these diseases, which include sickle-cell anemia and cystic fibrosis, cause mental retardation or death in early childhood. Both partners may appear normal, but by chance each carries the same harmful gene, in a recessive form. When they were conceived that defective gene was overpowered by a normal gene from one parent. Neither parent is aware that he or she carries the gene.

Unless they receive genetic counseling for some other specific reason, many couples will not discover that they are carriers until they give birth to an affected child. Fortunately, before pregnancy you can be checked with blood tests for certain severe recessive diseases.

Children will inherit the disease only if they receive the recessive gene from both parents. If you and your partner both carry the defective gene each child has a 25 percent chance of inheriting the birth defect. (Each child also has a 25 percent chance of inheriting two normal genes, in which case that child will be unaffected. And each child has a 50 percent chance of inheriting one normal gene and one recessive gene, in which case the child will appear normal but, like its parents, will be a carrier.)

No one knows how many recessive genetic defects there are; new ones are being discovered every day. Many inherited traits are simple characteristics like being able to wiggle your ears. But we do know that recessive-genetic diseases include several severe disorders.

Tay-Sachs Disease. If you are of Eastern European Jewish descent, genetic screening can uncover your risk for a metabolic disorder called Tay-Sachs disease, which results in fatal brain damage. The first signs of the disease may not appear until an infant is six months to a year old; then rapid decline in the functions of the brain and the nervous system lead to death, usually before four years of age.

Thanks to screening programs across the United States, Tay-Sachs has already been brought under control. Before pregnancy a blood test can determine whether one or both partners carry the gene. After pregnancy amniocentesis can detect Tay-Sachs disease in the fetus.

Sickle-Cell Anemia. Sickle-cell anemia, a disease affecting primarily blacks and Hispanics, stems from genetically defective hemoglobin, the protein in red blood cells that carries oxygen. In areas of the body where oxygen levels are low, this defective hemoglobin changes the normally disk-shaped cells to sickle-shaped cells.

The oddly shaped cells stick in capillaries and further reduce the delivery of oxygen, so that more and more cells "sickle." The usual 120-day life span of the blood cells is shortened, and as a result the person becomes anemic.

About 10 percent of American blacks are carriers and about one in every five hundred black infants is born with sickle-cell anemia. As circulation to various regions of the body becomes blocked, victims suffer attacks of severe pain. They also are vulnerable to infections, and such major parts of the body as the lungs, heart, brain, liver, kidneys, eyes, bones, and skin may be damaged. Modern treatment can help nurse afflicted children to adulthood, but no real cure has been found.

Before pregnancy a simple blood test can reveal if someone is a carrier. Until recently, however, there was no safety net for those couples who knew they might produce a child with sickle-cell anemia because no test could detect the disease in utero. As one woman put it, "Even when we turned the odds around and told ourselves that there was a three-in-four chance of having a healthy baby, it didn't seem worth the risk of having to watch your child suffer and die slowly."

A new prenatal procedure called fetoscopy offers some help for couples known to be carriers. Through fetoscopy samples of the fetus' blood can be withdrawn and examined for abnormalities. The test requires skill and delicacy; as fetoscopy becomes more generally available, genetic blood disorders like sickle-cell anemia will be more accurately diagnosed.

Thalassemia Major. If you or your partner are of Mediterranean ancestry, your blood may be tested before pregnancy for thalassemia major, or Cooley's anemia, another hereditary blood disease that can cause severe anemia in the baby. Afflicted children are seriously anemic and usually do not live past their early teens.

Thalassemia minor, also a genetic disease, produces a mild form of anemia and is not dangerous. However, two parents with thalassemia minor have a 25 percent chance of producing a child with thalassemia major. Like sickle-cell disease, until recently there has been no prenatal test to detect thalassemia in the fetus before birth. Fetoscopy, still relatively hard to obtain, is the first testing procedure for this disease.

Cystic Fibrosis. Cystic fibrosis is the most common inherited fatal disease among Americans, affecting about one out of every eighteen hundred live births. It is estimated, however, that about two thirds of children born with the disease die without it ever being properly diagnosed, leading some researchers to place the incidence of cystic fibrosis closer to one out of every thousand.

Affected babies are usually small at birth and may have an obstruction of the small intestine. Within the child's first year the first signs of lung damage may appear. Coughing bouts and frequent lung infections are common. A decade ago the average age of death was eight years. Today, with modern treatment, a child born with cystic fibrosis has a fifty-fifty chance of reaching age twenty-one. Some survivors are now living into their thirties and forties. This improved outlook has come about through early detection and persistent and aggressive therapy to prevent and treat the life-threatening respiratory complications.

In a recent breakthrough in trying to deal with this devastating disease, researchers in the United States, Canada, and England have succeeded in locating the cystic fibrosis gene from the huge morass of a cell's genetic material. Eventually, scientists may be able to isolate the gene, determine how it is abnormal, and correct or compensate for the abnormality.

For the present, an estimated ten million Americans unknowingly carry the gene for cystic fibrosis. Developing a simple, accurate means of detecting carriers before an affected child is born is one of the possibilities opened up by the recent genetic discoveries. Currently there is no reliable way to tell who has a hidden gene until and unless that person produces a child with cystic fibrosis. Anyone with a family history of cystic fibrosis is a potential carrier and should seek genetic counseling. If you are a suspected carrier, cystic fibrosis in a fetus can now be detected by a new test on amniotic fluid.

SEX-LINKED DISEASES

Of the twenty-three pairs of chromosomes in each cell, one pair determines sex. Females have two Xs; males have one X and one Y. An ovum always contains one X, and sperm may contain either an X or Y. Hence, it is always the father who determines the sex of a child.

Sex-linked genetic disorders occur only on one of the mother's X chromosomes and are passed down from mother to son. A female child born to a woman with an X-linked disorder has a 50 percent chance of becoming a carrier like her mother (the normal X she receives from her father dominates). A boy has a 50 percent chance of inheriting the defective X chromosome and, because he doesn't receive a protective normal X from his father, he will receive the disease itself.

There are 170 known X-linked disorders, most of them minor (color blindness is the most common, affecting about 8 percent of American men). But certain rare X-linked disorders are crippling. One of the most devastating is hemophilia, the bleeding disease. Another is Duchenne's muscular dystrophy, a disease usually fatal before the age of fifteen.

The family history reveals the odds. When there is a history of a severe sex-linked disorder in a family, pregnant women often choose amniocentesis to learn the sex of the fetus before birth. If the baby is a boy he has a 50 percent chance of inheriting the disease. The worst part about this is that if the couple chooses abortion, they may be aborting a healthy fetus. New fetal testing can help. Fetal blood sampling, via fetoscopy, can distinguish male fetuses affected by hemophilia from healthy male fetuses. In addition, families with sex-linked diseases may even have the option of choosing their child's sex *in advance of pregnancy* (see end of this chapter).

MULTIFACTORIAL DEFECTS

Most birth defects are caused by numerous genetic flaws interwoven with environmental factors. Neural-tube defects (NTDs), the second most common birth defect in the United States, fall into this category. These disorders are difficult for the genetic counselor to predict, but every day we are learning more about them.

Spina Bifida

Spina bifida is an NTD in which the bones of the spinal column do not fuse properly. In some affected infants the spinal cord protrudes outside the body through the opening in the spinal column. Spina bifida may be mild or severe. In its mild form the infant may have only slight physical disability; in its severe form the child may suffer severe disability, chronic illness, and mental retardation.

About one baby in two thousand is born with spina bifida or similar NTD disorders. Because the disease is the result of many genes interacting with one another or with environmental factors, your risk of having a baby with spina bifida is low, even if there is a history of the disease in your family. However, some genetic involvement is presumed because a family with one affected pregnancy has a 5 percent chance of a recurrence.

Before pregnancy, it's almost impossible for a genetic counselor to predict spina bifida. After pregnancy begins, however, fetal testing can detect the disease. Recent research has shown that the incidence of NTD is reduced when women are well nourished before conception and in the early weeks of pregnancy.

Cleft Lip and Cleft Palate

Perhaps most common of all the multifactorial defects are cleft lip and cleft palate, which occur in one out of every thousand babies. These defects occur because something happens to the fetus in its seventh week of development, and the upper portions of the fetal jaw fail to fuse correctly. Fortunately both can now be successfully corrected through surgery. Like all such defects, there is only a small risk that the disorder will recur in the same family. Cleft lip or cleft palate reappears in the same family about 2 percent of the time.

It's impossible to know what precisely has interfered with development, but certain drugs and viruses have been implicated. Sometimes cleft lip or cleft palate occurs as part of a larger group of more serious chromosomal abnormalities.

Other common birth defects caused by drugs or environmental factors include clubfoot, dislocated hip, and pyloric stenosis (a blockage of the stomach more common in boys than in girls), and heart defects. Surgery to correct these defects is usually successful: even with major defects of the heart or gastrointestinal tract, 75 percent of the children can be saved.

WHAT YOU CAN BE SCREENED FOR

Single-gene disorders are transmitted according to the basic laws of heredity and can be predicted in terms of odds for each child. Down's syndrome and spina bifida, on the other hand, are difficult to predict, as are environmentally caused defects.

If you have been exposed to a serious viral condition, abdominal X rays, or a teratogenic drug during early pregnancy, a genetic counselor can help you evaluate the amount of exposure and calculate the effects on the fetus. Likewise, if you are over age thirty-five, a counselor will advise you of the statistics that project the incidence of Down's syndrome in your age group.

TESTS DURING PREGNANCY

Even if you are at risk for transmitting a genetic disease, you may choose to become pregnant and through sophisticated new testing follow the growth of the fetus as it develops in the womb. Prenatal tests that directly—and indirectly—observe the development of the fetus are new, expensive, and not yet widely available. But they are a big step forward in the continuing search to prevent birth defects. Most available tests are now used to discover whether a fetus is handicapped, offering the parents the option of abortion. The future, however, promises that through such tests surgeons and geneticists may one day be able to correct birth defects while the fetus is still developing in the uterus. It is already possible in certain instances for babies to receive blood transfusions and other surgical procedures before birth.

Like genetic screening, however, prenatal testing for birth defects is only partially successful. Most birth defects *cannot* be diagnosed during pregnancy.

The most common prenatal tests performed today are ultrasound and amniocentesis. Yet other new tests are even more promising for the future.

Ultrasound Scans

An ultrasound scan uses pulsed sound waves which vibrate at high frequencies to obtain a picture of what is happening under water or inside a structure. Ultrasound was used during World War II to detect submarines and flaws in metal and it has been a diagnostic tool in obstetrics since the 1960s.

When directed into the uterus, some of the sound waves bounce off the baby's bones and other tissues; the echoes are converted into a black-and-white picture that builds up on a small television screen.

The procedure is simple and painless and usually takes only a few minutes. As you lie on your back, the doctor or radiographer covers your abdomen with a thin film of jelly or oil and passes a small device, called a transducer, back and forth across your abdomen. The picture that appears on the screen is difficult for the untrained eye to interpret, but the technician will explain it.

Although ultrasound is not the same as X ray, and is considered safe, it is used only for specific reasons during pregnancy. Obstetricians use the procedure to show the position and viability of the fetus and to reveal any gross abnormalities. Multiple pregnancies can be detected this way. Fetal growth can be monitored and ultrasound will show if the baby requires early delivery. Certain severe abnormalities, such as spina bifida, can be identified, as can problems affecting the heart, kidneys, and bowel. It is also sometimes possible to discover the baby's sex through ultrasound.

Ultrasound is commonly used to assist two other prenatal diagnostic tests, amniocentesis and fetoscopy.

Amniocentesis

Amniocentesis is presently the standard assessment of fetal health in women over thirty-five, women whose alpha fetoprotein (AFP) levels (see page 169) are elevated, or those who have a family history of certain birth defects.

Amniocentesis involves the removal of a small amount of the fluid from the amniotic sac surrounding the baby. Ultrasound is used first to locate the baby; after the procedure ultrasound is repeated to be sure the baby is unaffected. The physician administers a local anesthetic, then inserts a long thin needle through the abdomen into the amniotic sac and withdraws a small amount of amniotic fluid. The procedure takes only ten to fifteen minutes to perform and is not painful.

The fluid contains fetal cells, as well as protein, fats, enzymes, carbohydrates, hormones, and fetal urine, which makes it an ideal testing fluid. Cells in the fluid are grown, then examined under a microscope for abnormalities. Tests performed on the amniotic fluid can diagnose certain fetal defects and establish fetal maturity. Examination of the cells also reveals the baby's sex, which is important if there is a history of sex-linked disorders such as hemophilia or muscular dystrophy.

Amniocentesis is most often used to detect Down's syndrome, but more than a hundred different tests can be carried out on the fluid sample, each for a different birth defect. Amniocentesis carries only a small risk of miscarriage and is considered relatively safe, although the test is used only when there is reason to suspect a problem. The disadvantage of amniocentesis is that it cannot be performed until between the fourteenth and sixteenth week of pregnancy, and the results take up to four weeks to be known.

Chorionic Villi Biopsy

The prime advantage of this new test, chorionic villi biopsy, is the simplicity and speed with which it can be applied. Chorionic villi biopsy can detect birth defects between the eighth and twelfth week, much earlier than amniocentesis. Preliminary results, including whether Down's syndrome is present, are available within forty-eight hours; a thorough analysis comparable to that offered by amniocentesis takes two weeks.

The early testing provided by chorionic villi sampling means that if a woman decides to have an abortion she can do so in the first trimester. (An abortion after amniocentesis would take place in the less safe second trimester period.)

Despite its apparent advantages, researchers are concerned that since the test directly interferes with placental integrity, it holds greater risk of miscarriage. The miscarriage risk for chorionic villi biopsy is estimated between 1 and 2 percent, with some researchers putting it as high as 8 percent (compared with .05 percent for amniocentesis). But the test is so new that it has yet to be tested on a wide scale.

Presently a large controlled study comparing the safety of the two techniques is under way. If amniocentesis proves significantly safer, it may continue as the standard assessment for women over thirty-five. At that age, women tend to have more difficulty conceiving, and the press of time makes future pregnancies uncertain. Thus, older women or women with a history of infertility will wish to minimize as much as possible the risk of miscarriage. But if the major concern is to prevent the development of an abnormal pregnancy, then a slightly increased risk associated with chorionic villi testing may be worth taking.

The test takes about twenty minutes to perform; the physician inserts a thin tube, called an endoscope, through the mother's cervix up to the placental bed. The physician then guides a pair of special scissors through the endoscope and gently withdraws a small tissue sample from the chorionic villi, the finger-shaped protrusions on the chorion membrane surrounding the fetus.

Although the membrane is not actually part of the fetus, it does contain fetal tissue, so analyzing it can divulge a wealth of information. The test gives the same information as amniocentesis, including the gender of the fetus, and appears to offer the same degree of accuracy. Although the test is presently available in only a few hospitals, some researchers predict that the chorionic villi biopsy will replace many of the current uses of amniocentesis within the next several years.

Alpha Fetoprotein (AFP) Testing

AFP is a protein produced by the baby's liver which passes into the mother's blood via the placenta. When a woman is about sixteen weeks pregnant, her physician can take a routine blood sample and measure the AFP level in her blood. He or she expects to find a certain level of AFP in the sample, a sign that the fetus is developing normally. But a high level suggests a number of possibilities: a miscarriage may be threatening, or the mother may be carrying twins. Very high levels of AFP suggest that there may be a gap in the baby's skin that exposes the blood vessels, for example, in cases of neural-tube defects such as spina bifida. This is the primary reason for taking AFP levels.

The test is most accurate between the sixteenth and nineteenth week of pregnancy, although many doctors consider sixteen weeks the optimum time. If the level of AFP is high, the test is repeated on another blood sample. (An abnormally *low* level of AFP in the mother's blood may indicate Down's syndrome.)

If the second test is also abnormal, the fetus should be checked with an ultrasound scan, which can detect gross abnormalities, and possibly by amniocentesis to directly test the AFP level in the amniotic fluid surrounding the baby. These combined tests can detect about 85 percent of all babies with spina bifida. However, the accuracy of the tests can vary, and a raised AFP level does not necessarily mean a baby is abnormal.

Fetoscopy

Fetoscopy is a new, highly sophisticated procedure, in which the obstetrician inserts a long, fine fiber-optic telescope through the abdominal wall into the uterus for a direct look at the baby; the scope has a special channel through which the doctor can remove tiny samples of the baby's blood and tissue.

Fetoscopy is the only test that can determine the presence of certain crippling blood diseases or other severe birth defects, which means that it is invaluable when a couple is at risk to pass along sickle-cell anemia or thalassemia. If a woman is a known carrier of hemophilia, fetoscopy can determine whether a male fetus is affected. Because the procedure provides a direct look at the fetus, such defects as cleft palate and limb abnormalities also can be detected.

As with amniocentesis, a woman is usually given a local anesthetic, and the physician inserts the fetoscope into the abdomen with the guidance of ultrasound. Fetoscopy carries a higher risk of complications than other prenatal tests because the fetus is directly touched. The procedure is presently available in only a few hospitals. Fetoscopy is the only procedure that permits surgery to be carried out on the fetus.

In Utero Surgery
Only rarely can a birth defect be corrected while the fetus is still developing, but in those few instances fetoscopy is the procedure that allows lifesaving surgery to be performed. Two important operations can be carried out on the fetus: the first is a blood transfusion for a fetus that is severely anemic due to Rh-antibodies in its mother's blood (see Chapter 14); the other is to help a baby with a blocked urinary tract.

A blockage in the urinary tract causes a buildup of urine in the bladder, which can lead to irreparable kidney damage before birth. A blocked urinary tract can be discovered by ultrasound scan. Then surgery is carried out by threading a fine catheter through the mother's uterus into the bladder of the fetus. The fetal urine can then drain into the amniotic fluid as it should. The catheter remains in place until after the baby is born. After delivery, the tube is removed, and the blockage corrected by surgery.

Unfortunately not every fetus with a blocked urinary tract will benefit from this type of in utero surgery and the major problem is to select those who will. In the future it may be possible to perform bone marrow transplants and to provide treatment for thalassemia and other diseases via fetoscopy.

Ultrasound, amniocentesis, and fetoscopy can all reveal the baby's sex. If there is a possibility of a sex-linked hereditary disease you will obviously want to know the baby's sex. But if the tests are being carried out for another reason and you do not wish to learn the baby's sex in advance, tell your doctor beforehand.

CHOOSING THE BABY'S SEX BEFORE PREGNANCY

After the birth of their son three years ago, Marge and Donald Evans agreed that they wanted one more child and that it was to be a girl. Another couple with three girls arrived at the same conclusion, but they wanted a boy. Both couples got their wish through the use of a new gender-selection technique.

Over the centuries many theories have promised to control sex selection, ranging from timing of intercourse to using certain kinds of douches to eating certain kinds of foods. Even Aristotle, not known for flighty thinking, had a formula: make love in the north wind to conceive a male child and in the south wind for a girl.

More recent theories hold that the odds are skewed slightly in one direction or the other depending on the exact time of conception. Neither the ancient or more modern theories have proved reliable.

Now, a new artificial insemination technique that separates sperm into male and female cells claims to offer a 75 percent chance of correct selection. The technique is based on the theory that Y-carrying male sperm cells are faster swimmers than X-carrying female sperm cells. Sperm from the husband's semen sample are suspended in a cylinder of sticky albumin. The best swimmers reach the bottom of the cylinder first.

After two or three such swim-downs most of the sperm collected from the bottom of the cylinder (about 85 percent) are presumed to be Ys. These survivors are injected into the woman's cervix for artificial insemination.

The technique was developed by Dr. Ronald Ericsson, founder of Gametrics, which licenses the patented semen-filtering procedure to fertility clinics.

The new technique is still considered speculative by the medical community at large, but a recent study of over two hundred births that involved the procedure shows that it appears to raise the chances of having a boy to more than 75 percent. (The usual odds are slightly greater than 50 percent that a couple will have a boy in a given pregnancy. Worldwide, 106 boys are born for every 100 girls. Despite their slight advantage at birth, however, boys have a higher infant death rate, so girls soon outnumber boys.)

A slightly different technique is used to increase the chances of having a girl, and the success rate is reported to be about the same. However, several researchers caution that large-scale scientific tests are still needed to support the technique, and couples should approach it with caution.

If a sex-selection technique is perfected, it could have disturbing ethical and social consequences. Because parents requesting the technique have shown an overwhelming preference for male babies, would widespread use skew the national sex ratio?

One of the few studies on the subject comes from Dr. Roberta Steinbacher at Cleveland State University in Ohio and Dr. Faith Gilroy, at Loyolla College in Maryland. These social psychologists asked 236 women and men if they would use the method if it were available; about one quarter of them said they would. She then asked members of this second group which sex they would prefer; 81 percent of the women and 94 percent of the men said they would prefer their firstborn to be a boy. The reason most people gave for their choice was that boys had better opportunities in life than did girls.

Steinbacher worries that this overwhelming preference for firstborn males would, if openly acknowledged, undermine women's esteem. She suggests that the practice, if put in general use, would lead to a population of younger sisters that in turn might limit women to second-class status for the rest of their lives because of their ranking in the birth order. (Firstborns traditionally are considered to be achievers who tend to be more successful in school and careers than are siblings born later.)

This study was theoretical. In a later study Drs. Steinbacher and Gilroy asked women who were already pregnant whether they would prefer a boy or a girl, and the majority said they had no preference. Another study of two thousand couples who actually applied for the sex-selection technique found that nearly all of the couples who answered already had two or three children of the same sex and wished to limit the size of their family by having just one more child of the opposite sex.

Genetic Diseases
The desire to choose a baby's sex in advance could be especially important to couples who are carriers of certain sex-linked hereditary diseases such as hemophilia and muscular dystrophy. At least

two hundred such diseases have been identified and in the United States alone these are estimated to be responsible for several thousand deaths of newborn babies a year.

With preconception sex selection, a couple in which one partner had a family history of hemophilia might opt to have only female children since women, while they may be carriers of the gene, are not usually afflicted. Advocates of sex selection believe that the general population would eventually benefit by reducing the number of people suffering from such severe diseases.

As of now, genetic counselors do not routinely advise their clients who may carry sex-linked defective genes to try sex selection because sperm might be damaged while being handled outside the body.

Where does this leave us with sex selection? Are we looking into a future when such techniques would be banned because of the social implications? Or into a male-dominated future? Or into a future free of genetic defects?

As we ponder the ramifications, many couples are seeking the technique. The number of fertility clinics licensed to use the Gametrics procedure has doubled in the last six months, from eighteen to a total of thirty-six worldwide.

Modern genetics is on the threshold of discovery. While there is much to offer prospective parents in terms of pre-pregnancy screening, the real promise of genetics lies in the future.

On September 23, 1985, national guidelines were approved for a revolutionary type of medical treatment known as gene therapy to be used on humans against a range of fatal hereditary diseases. The treatment involves transplanting copies of normal genes into cells of a person whose own body lacks that gene or has it only in a malfunctioning form.

The approval clears the way for researchers to begin proposing specific therapies. The first diseases on which gene therapy is likely to be used are those involving a single gene. The patients most likely to benefit are those suffering from hereditary conditions that leave a person without normal immune defenses against infection and disease. In such cases cells might be removed from the afflicted person's bone marrow, modified, then reinserted.

In the future, scientists eventually hope to apply the techniques more broadly, and ultimately it is their hope that hereditary diseases will be eliminated.

CHAPTER 14

PREPARING FOR A
HIGH-RISK PREGNANCY

PHYSICIANS DISTINGUISH between high-risk and low-risk pregnancies in various ways. A low-risk mother is a woman in excellent general health, between the ages of eighteen and thirty-five.

Younger and older women are considered high-risk. So are women with a variety of problems, including malnutrition, venereal disease, drug abuse, smoking, and alcoholism. A woman who has had four or more children may have delivery problems, as might a woman who is unusually small in stature.

All of these women require special care during pregnancy, and their babies require skilled delivery. In this chapter, however, we're going to concentrate on women who have certain medical problems, such as diabetes and hypertension, that must be well controlled before they become pregnant.

Experts agree that more chronically ill women are choosing to have babies these days. Diseases that once killed women before they reached childbearing age are no longer routinely fatal, and technology has helped create a relatively new obstetrical specialty, maternal fetal medicine, that offers women sophisticated care by doctors committed to the success of their special pregnancies.

These doctors most commonly supervise pregnancies in women with diabetes, hypertension, heart or kidney disease, lupus, cystic fibrosis, or cancer. Because of advances in medical technology, the doctors say, the women rarely die during pregnancy or in childbirth. However, some pregnancies end with miscarriage, abnormalities in the baby, transmission of genetic disease, or deterioration of the mother's condition.

While some diseases, like cystic fibrosis, can worsen as a result of pregnancy, others go untreated and spread as a direct result of the pregnancy. This happens, for example, when a woman with cancer refuses chemotherapy or radiation that might harm the fetus. The specialist's role is to outline the risks of the pregnancy in detail and then, if the woman chooses to become pregnant, try to stabilize her disease before conception.

Early diagnosis of a preexisting disease, plus excellent control, are the keys to a healthy pregnancy. If you are on medication for a medical disease, you will want to discover if the drugs you take are safe during pregnancy. While the disease itself may be dangerous for the mother, the drug therapies often required for treating them are frequently hazardous to the unborn baby. There may be an alternative form of medication that you should switch to while you are pregnant. An important factor is strength of desire—a woman with a preexisting disease may have to severely alter her lifestyle, follow a more careful diet and, in general, be well-motivated to follow a regimen that will make pregnancy safe.

DIABETES

Out of every two hundred women who become pregnant, one is a diabetic. And four others will develop diabetes sometime during their pregnancy. Diabetes mellitus is the inability of the pancreas to secrete sufficient insulin to metabolize sugar. When blood sugar levels are elevated, the body cannot properly metabolize proteins, fats, and other nutrients. These and other changes in the metabolism of pregnant women can cause complications for the fetus.

High blood sugar levels in diabetic mothers are associated with severe congenital abnormalities and abnormally large babies who often die shortly after birth. If an overlarge baby survives, it often suffers serious medical complications. Before the discovery of insulin in 1921 diabetic women could rarely have a successful pregnancy. Today, with careful management, a diabetic woman has an excellent chance of having a healthy baby.

Two classes of medications are used to control diabetes: oral hypoglycemics and injections of insulin. The oral hypoglycemics should not be used during pregnancy, since animal studies have demonstrated a high incidence of fetal death and congenital anomalies with these agents. The treatment of choice for pregnant women is insulin, which has never been shown to produce abnormalities in humans. Further, insulin taken by a diabetic mother poses no hazards for breast-feeding. The insulin pump, which supplies a continuous flow of the hormone, has proved especially useful to pregnant women.

The diabetes should be controlled as well as possible with insulin and a good diet *before* conception because the demands of early pregnancy place an additional strain on a diabetic and the disease can easily go out of control.

During pregnancy, a diabetic woman must be closely monitored by an obstetrician who specializes in high-risk pregnancies, often in consultation with a specialist in diabetes. It is usual for a pregnant diabetic woman to see her doctor each week or two and have frequent checks made of her blood and urine sugar levels.

Your insulin dosage may have to be adjusted several times (insulin is usually increased during pregnancy). Further adjustments may be necessary if you travel. After the baby is born, insulin requirements usually return to pre-pregnancy levels. Throughout pregnancy, your obstetrician will vigilantly check for signs of urinary tract infection, preeclampsia, and any excessive accumulation of amniotic fluid around the fetus.

Working women with diabetes are usually able to continue work until early in the third trimester. However, if the diabetes is longstanding and severe, your obstetrician may advise you not to work at all during pregnancy.

Monitoring becomes even more painstaking during the final weeks of pregnancy. If prenatal tests show serious abnormalities, labor might have to be induced early. Unexplained stillbirth and overlarge babies are sometimes a complication of diabetes, and for this reason obstetricians often routinely advise delivery by cesarean section three or four weeks before term. Under various circumstances, however, a vaginal delivery might be feasible.

Gestational Diabetes
Diabetes that develops during pregnancy and disappears after the baby is born is called gestational diabetes. Women who are obese when they conceive or who have family members with diabetes are more likely to develop diabetes during pregnancy. You also have a

slightly increased risk if you previously gave birth to a baby weighing more than ten pounds; if you have had a stillborn baby or a baby with congenital abnormalities; if you have high blood pressure; if you are older than age thirty-five; or if you have traces of sugar in your urine.

The same risks apply as with regular diabetes: a risk that the baby will be overlarge and a risk of premature birth. Should you develop diabetes during pregnancy, early diagnosis and good medical care will help ensure delivery of a healthy baby. Initially, changing your diet may be enough to control the diabetes. But if blood and urine sugars cannot be controlled by diet alone you will need insulin. If you develop diabetes during pregnancy you have a 20 to 30 percent chance of becoming diabetic again later in life. To reduce your future risk, continue to exercise regularly after childbirth, eat a balanced diet, and maintain normal weight.

HEART DISEASE

Today many women with heart disease can successfully have children. Factors affecting the pregnancy are age and the extent of the disease process. The outcome is best if a woman is under age thirty-five, and if she has no history of heart failure and doesn't have to limit physical activity because of heart disease.

Women with heart disease often can have regular vaginal deliveries, although, to avoid the strain of the expulsive stage of labor, the baby is often assisted by forceps.

The drugs frequently prescribed to treat abnormal heart rhythms —digitalis and its derivatives and quinidine—do not appear to affect pregnancy, even though these agents pass freely from the mother's blood to the fetal circulation. Mothers who take quinidine, however, are usually advised not to breast-feed, since this drug passes into breast milk and may accumulate in the immature liver of a newborn.

HIGH BLOOD PRESSURE (HYPERTENSION)

During pregnancy blood pressure usually stays the same or temporarily decreases because of pregnancy hormones that relax blood vessels. For some women, however, high blood pressure may be present long before pregnancy or it may develop during pregnancy.

It's important to have your blood pressure checked *before* pregnancy to establish a base line. If your blood pressure is normal before pregnancy, but becomes elevated during pregnancy, it may be a warning sign of an impending problem (preeclampsia or toxemia). If your blood pressure is elevated before pregnancy, it can be brought under control with diet and/or medications before you conceive.

The cause of essential hypertension, which affects 5 to 10 percent of the adult population, is unknown. A slight degree of hypertension can often be controlled by diet and exercise, but most hypertensive people eventually have to receive drug therapy, which is lifelong. Without treatment, the disease leads to kidney failure, stroke, and heart attack. With adequate treatment, which reduces the blood pressure to safe levels, the hypertensive person leads a normal life.

Are the wide variety of antihypertensive agents used to control the disease safe for pregnant women? The answer seems to be that some are and some aren't. If you are being treated for high blood pressure you require careful evaluation, and possibly a change or adjustment in your medication before pregnancy. While most family physicians routinely treat hypertension today, you may wish to put yourself in the hands of a doctor who specializes in the treatment of high blood pressure simply because of the confusion about drug therapy and the many different kinds of drugs available. In addition, if your blood pressure is significantly elevated you may not be able to work during pregnancy.

Preeclampsia

High blood pressure is one symptom of a disease that occurs only in pregnancy, specifically after the twentieth week, called preeclampsia or toxemia. Most doctors agree that high blood pressure alone is not necessarily proof of the disease. Some women have high blood pressure in pregnancy without any other symptom and it doesn't develop into preeclampsia. The other classic symptoms of preeclampsia are rapid weight gain, fluid retention and swelling, and protein in the urine. Symptoms develop over a few days or may appear suddenly within twenty-four hours.

All pregnant women are screened for signs of preeclampsia at each prenatal visit. If preeclampsia is unnoticed and untreated it can develop into eclampsia, a dangerous condition which leads to convulsions and puts both the mother and baby at risk. Good nutrition, good prenatal care, and early treatment usually forestall these serious developments. Often a pregnant woman who develops preeclampsia requires bed rest in the hospital, as well as medication to bring the condition under control.

Edema and Salt

In the 1950s and 1960s excess salt was believed to contribute to the development of preeclampsia. In those days pregnant women were often treated with diuretics and given a low-salt diet to keep their weight and water retention down. It was eventually realized that eliminating salt can upset the important fluid balance in the body and that, in some instances, diuretics can damage a woman's kidneys and harm the fetus. New evidence suggests that inadequate consumption of protein is a more likely cause of edema.

Today, although there is still as much controversy about eating salt at any time, most obstetricians do not put their patients on salt-restricted diets to treat edema. Some slight edema is normal during pregnancy and a pregnant woman needs a certain amount of sodium to maintain a normal fluid balance in her body.

Swollen ankles during pregnancy are rarely a cause for concern. As the baby grows and the uterus expands the large vein that carries blood to the heart from the lower part of the body becomes constricted. The result is swelling in the lower part of the body. Often the only treatment necessary is to lie in bed on your left side, which prevents the uterus from pressing against that large vein, called the vena cava. Elevating your legs when sitting and wearing support stockings also helps. If these simple measures fail, and if edema becomes so severe that legs ache or hands become numb, your obstetrician may recommend a short course of diuretic therapy.

ALLERGIES AND ASTHMA

If you suffer from a persistent allergy, you should try to discover the cause before you become pregnant. The allergy may actually be a dietary deficiency or a side effect of smoking. If the condition persists after you give up smoking and improve your diet, you should consult an allergist.

Allergists usually begin with skin tests to find out which allergens are problematical for you. Ideally the allergy will be brought under control before you become pregnant—to avoid severe bouts and massive doses of medication during pregnancy.

There is some controversy about allergy treatment during pregnancy. Children born of allergic mothers are believed twice as likely as other children to develop allergies. Some doctors believe that their resistance is improved if their mothers continue to take allergy shots during pregnancy.

Allergy immunotherapy—a process by which a person periodically receives small injections of allergens to slowly build resistance to the offending agent—should be administered cautiously and only in minimal doses during pregnancy, especially during the first trimester.

Nasal Decongestants

It's common for pregnant women to suffer from nasal stuffiness and congestion, symptoms which usually disappear after delivery. Although the cause is unknown, doctors believe that pregnancy hormones are the culprits.

Medications to relieve such symptoms are so numerous and so commonly used that it's surprising that we don't know more about them. As it is, there is little information about the safety of these agents in pregnancy. Some studies have shown that certain antihistamines are statistically more likely than other agents to be associated with abnormalities in newborn babies, but many antihistamines and bronchial dilators are thought to be relatively safe to the fetus. The best advice seems to be not to use anything without first consulting your doctor. Even then, read the label of over-the-counter drugs and sprays carefully, and be alert for new labeling warnings.

Cortisone

Corticosteroids (cortisone) are invaluable in the treatment of severe attacks of bronchial asthma which are resistant to other forms of therapy, and medical reports indicate that some of these drugs are safe during pregnancy. However, corticosteroid users may encounter problems during labor, anesthesia, or surgery. The consensus of medical opinion seems to be that these agents should be used only when needed, and the pregnant woman should be carefully monitored for changes in blood sugar, sodium retention, and blood pressure.

SEIZURE DISORDERS

Anticonvulsant medications, while invaluable in the control of seizures, may increase the risk of fetal damage; but discontinuing the medication may cause even greater harm. If you suffer from a convulsive disorder, it's crucial that you have a full evaluation by a neurologist before becoming pregnant. If you have been free of seizures for several years, you may be able to discontinue medication during pregnancy. Or your physician may switch you to another drug with fewer risks to the fetus.

Studies suggest that the frequency of seizures stays the same in about half of pregnant women who suffer from convulsive disorders, and increases in 45 percent. Only 5 percent of pregnant women experience fewer seizures during pregnancy.

If your physician decides that you must take medication during pregnancy, follow his or her advice carefully. Severe and uncontrolled convulsions are more dangerous to both you and the baby than are the drugs. Your physician may even need to increase your regimen of anticonvulsant therapy during the course of pregnancy. If you require hydantoins or phenobarbital, you have an excellent chance of giving birth to a normal baby.

If you take anticonvulsants during pregnancy, your baby will receive an injection of vitamin K immediately following delivery to prevent bleeding. Afterward, the nursery staff will perform clotting factor and platelet counts periodically over the first twenty-four hours.

THE RHESUS FACTOR

Thanks to current medical prevention the rhesus, or Rh, problem is virtually a thing of the past. The Rh factor is a protein substance found on the surface of red blood cells, named for a similar substance found in the red blood cells of rhesus monkeys. Most people are Rh-positive, meaning that their red blood cells carry the Rh factor. About 15 percent of the population, however, do not have the Rh factor and are said to be Rh-negative.

The Rh factor is unimportant, unless you are Rh-negative and your baby is Rh-positive. During the course of pregnancy, some of the baby's red blood cells may seep into your circulation. Your immune system reads the unfamiliar protein on the blood cells as "foreign" and mounts an antibody reaction against them. These antibodies can invade the baby's bloodstream and destroy large numbers of its red blood cells.

Seepage is most likely to occur in late pregnancy or at delivery so there is little risk that a first pregnancy will be affected. But once the antibodies are established in your circulatory system they are ready to attack in full force any future pregnancy that is Rh-positive. Seepage of blood can also occur after an abortion, amniocentesis, or an ectopic pregnancy. Antibodies can also arise spontaneously.

When both partners are Rh-negative, the baby will also be Rh-negative, and no Rh problem can arise. Only when you are Rh-negative and your partner Rh-positive is there a potential problem. If this is the case, you should have a blood test before you become pregnant to find out if your blood already contains anti-Rh antibodies. If so, you are said to be Rh-sensitized; the sensitization is a permanent aspect of your immune system and a potential danger to future pregnancies. When this happens before pregnancy, some couples choose to have artificial insemination by a sperm donor who is also Rh-negative.

However, if you are not already sensitized to the Rh protein, the disease can be prevented. Blood tests are repeated after you conceive, then again later in pregnancy, and immediately after delivery to monitor sensitization.

Within seventy-two hours after delivery of your baby (and also after an abortion, amniocentesis, or an ectopic pregnancy—all situations in which the baby's red blood cells can seep into your circulation), you will receive an injection of Rhogam, which prevents your immune system from creating anti-Rh antibodies. Your blood continues to be free of antibodies and your next pregnancy is protected. The widespread use of Rhogam has dramatically reduced the incidence of severe anemia in Rh-positive babies.

Testing the Fetus
If blood tests show that a pregnant woman has a high antibody level, amniocentesis may be carried out to assess the condition of the fetus. If the test shows that many of the fetus's red blood cells

have been destroyed, labor may be induced or a cesarean section done. If the fetus is too immature to be born safely, it may receive intrauterine transfusions. Sometimes a fetus needs several transfusions before birth and may also need blood exchange transfusions after birth.

It is essential for a woman falling into any high-risk category to carefully prepare herself before pregnancy. This preparation includes a medical checkup with a specialist and possible adjustments in diet and medication. Preparation also means that the disease must be well controlled before she becomes pregnant.

There is one major risk category that affects an increasing number of American women: age. The chapter that follows offers a condensed view of the key medical issues facing women anticipating pregnancy after age thirty-five.

CHAPTER 15

PREPARING FOR PREGNANCY OVER AGE THIRTY-FIVE

IT'S NO LONGER NEWS that having babies later in life is a trend in the United States. While the overall national birthrate is down, the birthrate for women having their first child after age thirty has more than doubled. The 1983 report from the Bureau of the Census showed that childbirth for women bearing their first child after age thirty-five has increased dramatically in just three years, from 3.6 per 1,000 in 1980 to 5.2 per 1,000 in 1983.

Waiting to have children gives women certain advantages. The income and education level of women who delay childbearing usually improves. The Census Bureau report showed that 45 percent of recent mothers under thirty had family incomes under fifteen thousand dollars a year; only 14 percent had incomes above thirty-five thousand. New mothers over age thirty had a brighter financial outlook: only 27 percent lived in families with incomes below fifteen thousand dollars a year, and 40 percent had family incomes above thirty-five thousand.

A recent demographic study conducted by Judith Langer, president of a New York-based consumer research firm, found that older women having children for the first time were also more likely to be highly educated and established in professional occupations. Fully 45 percent of new mothers aged thirty and older are college graduates, compared with 12 percent of those aged eighteen to twenty-nine.

The primary difficulty with delayed childbearing is that the advantages do not coordinate with the biological facts. The most important thing to recognize is that the older you are, the more difficult it is to conceive. In terms of outward appearance women today age more slowly than did their own mothers and grandmothers. They look young and feel young well into middle age and beyond. But the biological processes that govern our reproductive lives tick relentlessly onward, regardless of how young we look.

Men, although their fertility declines somewhat after the age of forty, continue to produce millions of sperm daily throughout their lives. Although there has been some association between older fathers and birth defects, men generally can begin families at any age they choose. But many women who postpone childbearing get caught in a biological time warp: when we're ready, our bodies may not cooperate.

So the first thing an older woman has to recognize is that for a variety of reasons she may have difficulty becoming pregnant. The most fertile time for a woman is between age eighteen and twenty-eight. In this age group a woman has more than an 85 percent chance of becoming pregnant within one year when no contraceptives are used and when she has sexual intercourse on a regular basis.

From age twenty-eight on the reproductive cells (ova) begin to wind down. After age thirty every woman has a somewhat irregular pattern of ovulation, and her chances of pregnancy gradually diminish. After age thirty-five she has only about a 50 percent chance of becoming pregnant within one year—if the reproductive system is functioning perfectly. And things are less likely to be perfect at this age.

Many events may combine to decrease the odds: if a woman suffers from endometriosis, there is greater likelihood of increased tubal damage as she grows older, and there is a higher incidence of fibroid tumors of the uterus in older women. She has also had more time to encounter pelvic inflammatory disease and to have undergone surgery on the abdomen sometime during her life, two situations which may create scar tissue around the tubes. Fertility experts say that, all things considered, a woman over age thirty-five may have only a 25 percent chance of becoming pregnant.

CAN FERTILITY TREATMENT HELP?

If you wish to become pregnant but cannot conceive, should you seek help from a fertility expert? This is a difficult question to answer when a woman is over thirty-five. Fertility problems can be minor or severe. Few fertility problems are solved quickly—it usually takes several months for the problem to be diagnosed and treated, and even longer for positive results to occur. Many fertility specialists do not accept women over the age of forty because the chances of success are so slim.

By age thirty-five a woman's ovaries have begun to run out of eggs and, as a result, hormonal changes begin to take place on a subtle level. If a woman discovers in her mid to late thirties that her fallopian tubes are blocked, she can undergo surgery to correct the problem, but that doesn't increase the number of ova she has left.

However, if a woman's reproductive organs are healthy, fertility drugs such as clomiphene can be used to push the system and encourage existing ova to mature in the ovaries. Some fertility experts suggest that drug therapy can be used up to ages forty to forty-five. Because older women have an increased risk of giving birth to a child with Down's syndrome, amniocentesis is always recommended, although the fertility drug itself does not increase the risk of birth defects.

Menopausal Babies

Contrary to popular mythology, it is unlikely that you will become pregnant during perimenopause, the few years leading up to cessation of menses. The reason that some pregnancies take place so unexpectedly when a woman is in her late forties or even early fifties is that women approaching menopause do occasionally ovulate. But because they believe they are "menopausal" they have stopped using contraceptives.

A pregnant woman in this age group requires careful monitoring and delivery under the strictest, controlled conditions.

RISKS OF LATE PREGNANCY

When a woman does become pregnant after age thirty-five, however, her chances of delivering a healthy baby are very good, although she does require more careful monitoring by an obstetrician than does a younger woman. The dangers of late pregnancy are not nearly so great as is often believed. The likelihood of medical complications increases gradually, without sudden escalation, starting at about the age of thirty. The risk of pregnancy-related deaths (rising from eleven per hundred thousand in the late twenties, to eighteen in the early thirties, to forty-six in the late thirties) is small in any age group. After age thirty-five medical risks are still relatively low: nothing happens to a woman over thirty-five during pregnancy that doesn't also happen to younger women, but some problems occur with greater frequency. One of a woman's main concerns is her increased risk of giving birth to a child with a birth defect, particularly Down's syndrome.

Birth Defects
A woman has approximately four hundred thousand ova in her ovaries when she is born and each small reproductive cell has a limited life span. As you grow older, so do the ova. Certain birth defects, such as Down's syndrome, are associated with deteriorating chromosomes inside older ova.

The incidence of Down's syndrome rises from less than one per thousand before age thirty to one per hundred by age forty. Even so, women over thirty-five have a good chance of having a normal baby.

Some fetal abnormalities can be detected early in pregnancy with new prenatal tests (amniocentesis or chorionic villi biopsy) that can detect Down's syndrome as well as certain other chromosomal defects. Because abortion is an option, older women need first to resolve some pressing issues. Will they have amniocentesis to detect Down's syndrome? If the test indicates that the child will be defective, will they choose abortion? (If the fetus does have Down's syndrome, the odds greatly favor a second normal pregnancy.)

The question of what to do about a defective fetus should be resolved before the woman becomes pregnant, and husband and wife need to make the decision together.

Birth defects, however, are only one concern of the older woman. Her own health and her ability to carry the child to term are also cause of concern.

Complications During Pregnancy

The primary risk for older women is spontaneous abortion. Spontaneous abortion in the first three months of pregnancy occurs 3.5 times more frequently in women over thirty-five than in younger women. This increased frequency is believed to be due to chromosomal abnormalities.

Other pregnancy complications include stillbirths, placenta previa, diabetes, and high blood pressure. Multiple births also occur more often with increasing age—a woman in her thirties has a 30 percent greater chance of having twins than she did in her twenties.

Many of the risks of postponed pregnancies are related to preexisting medical conditions such as diabetes, kidney disease, hypertension, cardiovascular problems, and uterine fibroids (see Chapter 13). Although these illnesses are more common among older people, your chances of developing one of them are relatively small.

For any woman the most dangerous risk in pregnancy is preeclampsia (toxemia)—a dangerous form of edema which can lead to convulsions in the mother and death to the fetus. The incidence of preeclampsia triples in women under age twenty and over age forty, but again even if signs should appear, good medical care prevents progression of the disease. As a precaution, all pregnant women are screened for signs of preeclampsia at each prenatal visit. The symptoms, which typically arise late in pregnancy, include increased blood pressure, excess fluid retention, rapid weight gain, and protein in the urine.

Delivery Problems

An older woman having her first child is also more likely to have problems during delivery. The cervix may not dilate properly, and there is more likelihood of prolonged labor and hemorrhage. All of these problems can be handled in a well-equipped modern medical facility.

Cesarean delivery, which bypasses some of these problems, requires major abdominal surgery and is not considered necessary for most older mothers. Natural delivery usually puts less stress on a woman's body than a cesarean section. Most obstetricians today agree that if an older woman can deliver naturally, she should be allowed to do so. The obstetrician watches her closely and monitors her progress by pelvic exam and fetal assessment. If everything progresses normally, the baby should be born without complications. The primary danger during delivery is that the placenta may be misplaced or the blood vessels may collapse. These events happen quickly. The moment anything out of the ordinary occurs, the obstetrician indicates a cesarean delivery.

A cesarean section is usually scheduled beforehand if fetal monitoring shows that the blood flow to the placenta is deficient, or if the fluid starts to prematurely leak out of the amniotic sac.

GETTING READY

Is there anything you can do ahead of time to get in shape for a postponed pregnancy? The keys to enhancing a late pregnancy are early and conscientious obstetrical care, good nutrition, and genetic counseling. By the time you reach age thirty-five, your body has gone from a protein-building system to a system of simple replacement.

Pregnancy places great demands on your whole body at any age. For the older woman the extra weight of pregnancy is distributed on joints less limber than those of a younger woman. Low back pain and arthritic changes in the knees are not unusual.

Pregnancy also accelerates cell metabolism, which means that disease processes may speed up. For example, pregnant women at age thirty-five have a greater tendency to develop diabetes.

It is especially important for an older woman to get in good physical shape before pregnancy. In addition to a good nutrition plan, you need to work out an exercise program designed to strengthen the lower back and muscles of the abdomen. Jogging is not the best way for older women to get in shape for pregnancy. Jogging can injure knee joints and also tends to decrease weight, which may interfere with ovulation. An aerobic program will tune up all the body functions. Overall, swimming is probably the best exercise for older women looking forward to pregnancy. The pre-pregnancy exercises described in Chapter 11 are especially helpful for older women because they address the specific areas of the body that most need to be strengthened.

The hardest part of childbirth for older women is becoming pregnant. If you conceive, the key to a successful pregnancy is good diet, daily exercise, and careful prenatal observation. As soon as you become pregnant, your obstetrician can begin to test your system for early signs of such medical problems as elevated blood sugar, which suggests diabetes. The obstetrician will watch you closely throughout pregnancy.

Whether you should wait until you are older to have children can be decided only in the context of your life in general. If your personal, social, and emotional needs tell you that you should wait, then it is probably better to wait, even though there is a somewhat higher risk of complications with a late pregnancy. But it's also true that more than 95 percent of women over thirty-five have healthy babies with few complications.

CHAPTER 16

IF YOU HAVE HAD
A MISCARRIAGE

IF YOU HAVE HAD one or a series of miscarriages, what are your chances of a normal pregnancy? What steps can you take to prepare yourself to ensure a healthy pregnancy the next time you conceive?

Early spontaneous abortion or miscarriage is so common that many physicians consider it a natural part of genetic selection. The Centers for Disease Control in Atlanta estimates that 10 to 20 percent of all pregnancies abort naturally, most often before the twelfth week, and many of these go completely unnoticed. Although exact statistics do not exist, recent studies suggest that the figure may actually be as high as 30 to 50 percent.

Despite these statistics, many physicians do not consider miscarriage a serious medical problem. The cause of the miscarriage is often untraceable, usually attributed to the accidental fusion of an abnormal ovum or sperm. After one miscarriage few doctors advise any special investigation or tests, unless the miscarriage occurred late in pregnancy, because a single miscarriage is usually followed by successful pregnancy. After the loss of one pregnancy, the statistical chance of a successful second pregnancy is more than 80 percent.

Risk of repeated miscarriage increases only if a specific cause, such as a hormonal problem, is present. In that case, chances of a successful pregnancy are slim unless the cause is identified and treated.

If you've had two miscarriages, or you have a family history of birth defects, most physicians would recommend a physical and genetic evaluation. Some specialists today believe that every miscarried or stillborn fetus should receive meticulous genetic testing. During the next pregnancy, they also might suggest amniocentesis and ultrasound scans to follow the development of the fetus. There is no hard-and-fast rule about the best time after a miscarriage to try to conceive again. Physically, waiting for three to six months is what most doctors suggest. Emotionally, only you can know when you're ready to try again. Miscarriage at any stage of pregnancy can be a devastating experience, and it's important to allow yourself time to recover emotionally before trying again.

RISK FACTORS

Even though miscarriage can be caused by several different factors and in many cases the cause is unknown, some specific risk factors have been identified. If you can identify one or more of these risk factors even after one miscarriage, it might be possible to prevent another one.

Possible Causes

Miscarriage or spontaneous abortion refers to the loss of the fetus before the twenty-eighth week of pregnancy. (After this, miscarriage is called premature labor.) Contrary to movies and popular mythology, miscarriage is almost never caused by physical exertion, unless there is already something wrong with the pregnancy. The well-cushioned fetus is firmly attached to the inside of the uterus and virtually impossible to dislodge. Running, jogging, swimming, and other sports have not been shown to initiate miscarriage.

The two most common causes of early miscarriage are abnormal development of the fertilized ovum and incorrect implantation of the embryo in the lining of the uterus. These causes may be isolated —occurring one time only—or they may be the cause of repeated miscarriage.

Advanced maternal age and smoking are known risk factors. So are venereal disease and a history of pelvic inflammatory disease which can lead to ectopic pregnancy.

Other contributing causes include general illness, infections that involve the lining of the uterus, high blood pressure, or kidney disease. Certain environmental pollutants have also been linked to chronic miscarriage (see Chapter 7).

WHEN MISCARRIAGE THREATENS

Impending miscarriage sometimes presents warning symptoms in time for the pregnancy to be saved. Bleeding or spotting signals a threatening abortion. Some miscarriages are completely painless, therefore any vaginal bleeding during pregnancy, even if there is no pain, should be immediately reported to your doctor. Although the pregnancy may be in danger, the chances that it will continue are good.

The treatment to prevent a miscarriage depends on the type of miscarriage and the approach of the physician. The most common treatment is bed rest. Whether or not a threatening abortion stabilizes with bed rest appears to have more to do with the nature of the problem than with physical exertion. Recent studies show that physical stress seems to play only a minor role in miscarriage. However, when bleeding and cramping signal an impending abortion, the physician usually will put the patient to bed for a few days in the hope that the embryo will settle itself into the uterus. The cramping may halt, and the pregnancy then proceeds normally.

If this happens to you, you needn't worry that with bed rest you have saved a defective embryo. When a threatening abortion recovers and the pregnancy successfully reaches term, the chances are excellent that the baby is normal.

A threatening abortion may advance to an inevitable abortion that cannot be halted. More than half of all miscarriages in the first trimester are due to genetic defects in the embryo, and these pregnancies cannot be saved. Bleeding becomes intense, painful contractions cause the cervix to dilate, the neck of the womb opens up, and the embryo passes out. If the abortion is complete, pain ceases, bleeding subsides, and the uterus firmly contracts.

If any bits of tissue remain inside the uterus, the miscarriage is termed incomplete. This is a dangerous condition that requires a dilation and curettage (D&C) within a few hours of the event to scrape all remnants of the tissue out of the uterus.

Sometimes a woman will have a missed abortion, in which the fetus dies in the uterus but is not expelled. Labor can be induced or a D&C performed to evacuate the uterus. It's estimated that a missed abortion occurs once in every hundred pregnancies.

Warning Signs

If your pregnancy has been confirmed, or if you have missed a period and suspect you are pregnant, see your doctor as soon as possible if you experience any of these symptoms:
Abdominal cramps
Severe abdominal pain, followed by bleeding
Slight spotting or staining of dark blood
Dizziness
Pain in the shoulder, which may be "referred" pain from the abdomen.

ECTOPIC PREGNANCIES

An ectopic pregnancy is one in which the fertilized ovum does not complete its journey to the uterus and implants in one of the fallopian tubes; occasionally it may start to grow within the mother's abdominal cavity. Ectopic pregnancies are dangerous; they always result in the loss of the embryo and sometimes risk to the mother's life.

An ectopic pregnancy can happen to any woman at any age, but the risk increases among women over age thirty-five. Endometriosis or mechanical obstructions inside the fallopian tubes are definite contributing causes, although the embryo may be misplaced even when the reproductive organs are completely normal.

The number of ectopic pregnancies has tripled in the last ten years, reaching a peak of 52,200 in 1980. One outstanding factor accounts for this dramatic rise: the recent increase in PID, traceable to such sexually transmitted diseases as gonorrhea and chlamydia. Even when treated early and successfully, PID can leave behind strictures and scarring inside the fallopian tubes that block the passage of a fertilized ovum into the uterus. Women with a history of PID are seven times more likely than others to have ectopic pregnancies.

The major concern is that the pregnancy will rupture before the condition is diagnosed. Early warning signs—cramps and spotting beginning around the eighth to tenth week of pregnancy—are easily overlooked. The next warning sign is more bleeding and more severe pain.

These symptoms are easily confused with a simple miscarriage or with such other emergencies as appendicitis or pelvic inflammatory disease. A pregnancy test at this time may be positive or negative, depending on whether the embryo is still alive. Ultrasound, and sometimes laparoscopy, is needed to confirm the diagnosis. Once an ectopic pregnancy is located, it must be quickly removed by surgery under a general anesthetic. Delay can result in rupture, followed by severe hemorrhaging. Surgical intervention can save the woman's life and also preserve the reproductive organs. An ectopic pregnancy may implant anywhere within the interior of the fallopian tube, sometimes lodging on the very end of the tube and attaching to the ovary. Often one fallopian tube, and sometimes an ovary, must be removed. New laser surgery can often preserve both tube and ovary.

If the ectopic pregnancy is caused by an obstruction in the fallopian tube, the risk of another ectopic pregnancy is high unless the blockage is removed and the tube reconstructed. Unfortunately the surgery to rebuild the tube often creates more scar tissue. If you require this delicate tubal reconstruction, select a highly skilled microsurgeon, and consider laser microsurgery, a technique that appears to reduce postsurgical scarring.

When the ectopic pregnancy is caused by other accidental factors, the event may never recur and, if the fallopian tubes can be preserved, a woman has a good chance to have a normal pregnancy in the future. Generally, if a woman experiences repeated ectopic pregnancies in the same fallopian tube, physicians recommend the removal of that tube in order to prevent damage to the ovary. In that case, fertilization can still take place in the other tube, or the woman may be a candidate for in vitro fertilization.

INCOMPETENT CERVIX

Normally, the cervix remains closed until labor begins, then it dilates to allow the baby to be born. But sometimes the cervix is naturally weak or has been weakened by injury during a D&C or previous childbirth. As the fetus grows larger, the incompetent cervix is unable to sustain the increased weight; it dilates prematurely and the pregnancy falls out. An incompetent cervix is a major cause of a second trimester miscarriage.

An incompetent cervix seldom can be spotted before the fact. The way most women learn they have the condition is that they have repeatedly sustained painless miscarriages after the twelfth week of pregnancy. However, once the condition is identified, it can be treated. When an obstetrician knows that a pregnant woman has an incompetent cervix, he can place a stitch around the cervix to tighten it and support the pregnancy.

If this procedure, called the Shirodkar suture, is performed early enough, the woman has an 80 percent chance of a successful pregnancy. The stitch is removed shortly before term; if labor starts early, the stitch is removed immediately.

PREMATURE LABOR

By definition, premature labor occurs after the twenty-eighth week of pregnancy and before the thirty-seventh week. Complications of prematurity account for 90 percent of all babies who die just before, during, or soon after delivery.

Risk factors include poor prenatal care and anemia. Women under twenty years of age, heavy smokers, and those who are undernourished are also at greater risk.

Often there is no apparent reason for premature labor. It may, however, be caused by premature rupture of the fetal membranes; a multiple pregnancy; an excess accumulation of amniotic fluid; an incompetent cervix; or maternal infections, especially urinary tract infection.

Occasionally premature labor begins after a fright or a sudden emotional disturbance, but it's difficult to know whether such a sequence of events is the true cause or merely a coincidence.

When a woman suffers a premature delivery, it's important to try to discover the reason. Some problems can be surgically corrected; problems caused by diabetes or other illnesses can be medically treated during pregnancy.

STILLBIRTH

A child that develops to term but dies just before delivery is called a stillbirth. Stillbirth occurs when for any reason the flow of oxygen from the mother to the baby is cut off. Oxygen can be blocked in several ways: blood clots may form in the umbilical cord, or the placenta may pull away from the baby prematurely. Both of these events usually occur within the last few weeks of pregnancy. The classic symptom is that the mother no longer feels the infant moving inside her womb. Labor is induced as quickly as possible to reduce emotional stress and potential medical complications.

In some cases, the umbilical cord may become trapped and compressed during delivery, and the baby's air supply is cut off. Today such entanglements are detected with fetal monitoring, and the child can be delivered by cesarean section or other emergency obstetrical maneuver.

MULTIPLE LOSSES

Women who sustain three or more miscarriages are termed chronic aborters. The problems associated with chronic abortion are numerous, complex, and only partially understood, and experts seldom agree. The cause may lie with the woman or with her husband. With any woman who repeatedly aborts, the couple needs to find a fertility specialist who is willing to aggressively pursue the problem until it is solved.

Repeated miscarriage may be caused by hormonal problems, uterine growths, fibroid tumors, an incompetent cervix, or a misshapen uterus, all problems that can be surgically corrected. For repeated early abortion linked to inadequate development of the endometrium, some doctors give injections of progesterone to build the uterine lining. The benefit of hormone treatment is still speculative.

About 7 percent of couples where women sustain multiple abortions have a chromosome problem, and genetic testing will reveal the problem. Genetic specialists believe that every miscarriage or stillborn fetus should receive meticulous laboratory evaluation, including X rays and karyotyping. Many hospitals today routinely perform genetic testing on aborted fetuses.

THE EMOTIONAL AFTERMATH OF MISCARRIAGE

If you have miscarried in the past, one of the most important things you will have to face before becoming pregnant again is the emotional trauma. The death of a child before birth is a loss whose severity is rarely recognized by family and friends and sometimes not by the husband and wife themselves. The couple grieves for a

loved one whose existence was evanescent, a child who was anticipated but never actually seen. Because of the ambiguous nature of
miscarriage, the couple often is not able to resolve one loss before
being faced with another. Trying to quickly get over the loss usually
makes the grieving process more difficult.

Psychologists feel it helps to recognize the universal stages of
grieving that we all experience when anyone close to us dies. Only
after the initial feelings of numbness begin to pass are couples generally ready to openly express their grief. Unfortunately this is the
time that family and friends often assume that they've gotten over
their loss. Even couples who lose a baby early in pregnancy have
come to see themselves as parents and may experience many weeks
of sadness and crying.

There is often strain on a marriage after a miscarriage, particularly
if the partners deal with their grief at different paces. But the biggest
problem is often friends who don't know what to say, and hospital
staff who tend to act as if nothing happened.

Three years ago Lisa Jenner lost a son in her seventh month of
pregnancy. One day the child simply stopped moving. At the hospital labor was induced and the baby was stillborn. Afterward she
recovered in a room on the maternity floor where new mothers were
nursing and cuddling their babies. "The nurses and doctors acted as
if nothing was wrong. The message I got from them was not to talk
about what had happened." Weeks after Lisa went home, she still
suffered bouts of weeping and depression.

During the months that followed, Lisa and her husband, Todd,
were lucky enough to find comfort from their neighbors next door
who had also lost a child. They joined an informal support group,
one of several which today meet regularly in major cities around the
United States. Thanks to the efforts of such groups there is a changing attitude toward miscarriage and stillbirth. Couples are less likely
to accept assurances that all was for the best and are more likely to
grieve openly for a time rather than sweep the memories away.

SHARE, at St. John's Hospital (800 East Carpenter Street, Spring-
field, Ill. 62769), is a clearinghouse for support groups for couples
the woman of which has suffered miscarriage or stillbirth. It lists
328 groups across the country. Through the groups, parents learn
that it is all right to refuse invitations to visit friends with children,

and that it is common to blame themselves even though they know they've done nothing wrong.

The medical profession is changing also, as parents become less accepting of the platitude "That's nature's way," and physicians are more aggressively seeking the cause behind even a single miscarriage. Learning as much as possible about the cause of the miscarriage can give the couple something real to hold on to in a very unreal situation. If the fetus is aborted early, laboratory tests can be performed, particularly chromosome analysis, to try to identify the cause of the miscarriage.

In the wake of the network of parent support groups a few hospitals have organized bereavement programs. Staff members at these parent-sensitive institutions encourage couples to see and hold their infant if it was fully formed and to arrange a funeral or memorial service. They talk to couples about their loss and are trained to treat the miscarriage like a death, not a secret.

It's important to work through these feelings before attempting another pregnancy. But some couples must try for another pregnancy, even while they are still mourning, to stay ahead of the steadily ticking biological clock. Support from friends and other couples whose pregnancies miscarried can help them work through the loss and decide when enough time has passed to try again. It is reassuring to know that following one or even two miscarriages there is a 70 percent probability of successful pregnancy.

CHAPTER 17

HELP FOR
INFERTILE COUPLES

THE WIDE PRESS COVERAGE of the infertility epidemic has alarmed many
couples, especially those who have postponed childbearing until
their thirties. Once they decide to have a baby they often become
anxious if the woman doesn't become pregnant immediately.

Statistics confirm that their concern may be justified. In the past
twenty years the incidence of infertility in the United States has
nearly tripled, so that today one in five American couples is desig-
nated as infertile. This is a rapidly climbing statistic and some new
research predicts that this figure will soon reach one couple in three.

Since infertility usually has no symptoms—no pain or headaches,
no pulled muscles or broken bones—it's impossible for nonconceiv-
ing couples to know whether they actually have a fertility problem
or whether the mathematical odds are simply running against them
for the time being. If you are unable to achieve pregnancy right
away, how soon should you start to worry about fertility?

According to fertility expert Dr. Joseph H. Bellina, director of the
Omega Institutes in New Orleans and adviser to the Child and Human Development Council of the National Institutes of Health, if
you're feeling worried, it's time to consider professional consultation. Most people, says Bellina, have an instinctive notion of
whether or not they should have conceived a child. If you are worried, ask an expert.

The first person to consult is your family physician or gynecologist, who will tell you whether you're too concerned too soon. Usually an office visit and a brief discussion will put you on the right
track.

In general, any couple who has been actively trying to have a baby for a year or longer may be candidates for professional counseling. If you know that you have certain risk factors—for women, a history of pelvic infection, missed periods, or menstrual pain; for men, scrotal injuries—you may seek counseling even earlier. Women over the age of thirty should probably seek counseling if they haven't become pregnant within six months.

Doctors place much of the blame for the epidemic on the spread of venereal disease, particularly chlamydia and gonorrhea, which in women has led to an increasing occurrence of pelvic inflammatory disease. Since statistics about male infertility were not kept in the past, it is unknown if the incidence of infertility in men is also rising or if it has remained steady.

Today infertility is about equally divided between women and men. About 30 percent of the time the problem can be traced to the female, and 30 percent of the time to the male partner. In another 30 percent, *both* partners will have a fertility problem. Unfortunately, for 10 percent of all infertile couples, no known cause can be discovered.

Because of the overlap between men and women, both partners should participate in a fertility evaluation. A complete workup demands a wide range of tests and investigations. And because both partners may have more than one problem, all related tests are usually performed to make sure nothing is missed. Each partner begins the workup with a medical history and physical examination, followed by specific fertility tests.

INFERTILITY IN WOMEN

Occasionally a woman is infertile because something may have happened during fetal development or childhood, but most causes of infertility arise in adult life. Fertility problems in adult women are divided almost equally into two fairly distinct categories. The first category, called ovulatory failure, has to do with ovulation.

Ovulation Problems

At least half the fertility problems in women are attributed to ovulatory failure. The egg may not mature properly; or if it does grow, it may not release from the ovary on schedule. The operation of the ovaries is overseen by the hormonal axis that runs between the brain, the pituitary gland, and the ovaries. If this axis is even slightly disturbed, the system can misfire and ovulation won't occur. Some errors occur spontaneously in the timing mechanism of the hormonal axis. Others are perpetrated by illness or drugs, particularly the birth control pill. It's not unusual for a woman to have trouble resuming her normal pattern of ovulation after stopping the pill. Generally this condition cures itself within a few months but, occasionally, medical treatment is needed to reestablish the system.

Modern fertility drugs that manipulate the pathway between the hypothalamus and the pituitary gland can solve many ovulatory problems. The drug clomiphene can induce ovulation in nearly 80 percent of all women with ovulatory failure. Clomiphene acts directly on the hypothalamus, forcing it to boost the pituitary, which in turn drives the ovaries to produce and release eggs. When clomiphene fails, the extremely potent Pergonal may work. Pergonal, which has the potential for severe side effects, requires careful monitoring.

Blocked Tubes and Other Mechanical Problems

The second major category of fertility problems for women involves "mechanical" failures in which the reproductive organs themselves are damaged. Twenty years ago blocked tubes, pelvic adhesions, and other obstructions accounted for only about 25 percent of infertility in women. Today that figure has jumped to more than 40 percent. The major reason behind the soaring incidence of mechanical infertility is infection in the pelvic cavity, called pelvic inflammatory disease. (See Chapter 9.)

Such infections, primarily venereal disease, usually reach the pelvic cavity via sexual intercourse. Scars or adhesions form from the debris left behind by white blood cells which swarm over the foreign bacteria in an effort to destroy the infection. Rapid treatment can stop massive damage, but even a little scar tissue in the wrong place can interfere with pregnancy.

Another major cause of scar tissue and adhesions within the pelvic cavity is endometriosis, a painful and destructive disease in which bits of the endometrial lining of the uterus begin to grow in various sites throughout the abdomen. How the endometrial tissue escapes from the interior of the uterus is unknown; but somehow the cells implant on the outside of the uterus and on the ovaries or bowel and continue to grow just as if they were inside the uterus. Every month the implants, stimulated by the same hormones that build the endometrium of the uterus, grow and spread throughout the pelvic cavity. At the end of the monthly cycle the tissue bleeds just like the endometrium, and bleeding creates scar tissue. Remnants of the misplaced tissue burgeon again the following month. The disease can spread through the pelvic cavity until the ovaries and tubes are smothered in scar tissue.

About 15 percent of all women have endometriosis, and the incidence of infertility among them is nearly 50 percent. Although endometriosis can occur at any age, it occurs most frequently in women over thirty who have never had children. As more and more women delay childbirth, the incidence of infertility related to endometriosis is likely to increase. If a woman with endometriosis can become pregnant in her early twenties, she may avoid the worst repercussions of the disease.

Treatment for endometriosis, although complex and lengthy, is often successful. It may include surgery or drugs, or both, and physicians disagree about a standard approach. Treatment usually depends on the extent of the disease, as well as the woman's age. There are good arguments for both medical and surgical treatment, and the success rate for combined treatment is good.

Any surgery performed on the abdomen can also create scarring around the reproductive organs, particularly if the operation was complicated by infection. Women who had appendectomies when they were children are often surprised to discover years later that they are infertile as a result.

Microsurgery
Karen, a twenty-four-year-old teacher from Iowa learned from a laparoscopy (a view inside the abdomen via a long, slender telescope inserted through the umbilicus) that her whole pelvic cavity was sheeted in thick scar tissue. When Karen was four years old she had undergone an emergency appendectomy, which was complicated by severe infection. She had no idea that as a result massive scar tissue had enveloped all of her reproductive organs.

A few years ago her situation would have been hopeless. The reproductive organs are small and delicate, difficult to see, and virtually impossible to operate on in the conventional manner. When the microscope was used in surgery, surgeons were no longer limited to what they could see with their own eyes. Microsurgeons today can rebuild a damaged fallopian tube by nicking out the blockage, then matching up and neatly stitching together the layers of the tube. Even microsurgery couldn't help Karen, however. But a more recent advance, the surgical laser, could. A skilled microsurgeon used the precise carbon dioxide laser to etch out and free the reproductive organs from the massive adhesions that bound them together in a solid block. In this particular case, because the damage was so extensive, Karen was given only a 25 percent chance of pregnancy. Without surgery, however, her chances were zero.

The surgical laser reduces one of the major pitfalls of traditional surgery—new scarring caused by the corrective surgery itself. Because the laser causes less damage to the surrounding tissue, less bleeding, and requires fewer sutures, it usually creates less scar tissue during the healing process. Laser surgery, which cuts and seals tissue in one motion, also reduces the operating time, which means that less anesthetic is needed.

Cervical Problems
A third, less frequently seen group of problems involves the route traveled by sperm as they swim from the vagina through the cervix and uterus and into the tubes. Problems here may originate during fetal development when, for various reasons, the uterus or vagina may not have formed properly. About 80 percent of these birth defects can be corrected with surgical reconstruction.

Between 10 and 15 percent of fertility problems in women involve the cervix, which must produce good-quality mucus to provide a proper environment for sperm, and the uterus, which must be in good shape to allow for implantation and proper growth of the fertilized egg. Should even a mild infection set in, the cervix can produce a hostile, killing mucus that destroys sperm on contact. In the uterus, a rare inflammation of the endometrium, called chronic endometritis, can interfere with implantation of the ovum. Both conditions can be treated with antibiotics; occasionally a D&C is needed to remove endometrial tissue.

Aging

Although aging has little effect on male fertility, a woman's most fertile years are between the age of eighteen and twenty-eight, when ovulation is most regular. Also, as has been mentioned, ova, which are present at birth, begin to deteriorate and lose some of their capability for fertilization as a woman ages. So by the time she reaches menopause a woman's supply of ova is depleted. If her husband has a slightly lowered sperm count, together they may be infertile. (See Chapter 15.)

The Environment

Many elements outside the body influence what is going on inside. For example, a new study has shown conclusively that fertility is impaired among women who smoke. Exercise also may be a cause of temporary infertility. Women who exercise strenuously or those who experience dramatic weight loss often stop menstruating, a sign that ovulation has ceased. But new research on exercise shows that even those women whose menstrual cycles appear normal may not be ovulating regularly.

Men are also subject to environmental stress. Heat, altitude, and drugs, to mention only a few, can all affect sperm production in men. As sperm cells grow and mature they become increasingly sensitive to toxic agents from the environment.

Psychological Factors

Not so long ago thousands of women were told that their inability to conceive was strictly mental. Modern science has shown that the vast majority of these women probably had undiagnosed physical problems that caused their infertility. In fact, today 90 percent of all cases of infertility can be accurately diagnosed, compared with only 40 percent ten years ago. Many researchers in the field are so impressed with these advances that they believe they will eventually be able to identify a physical cause for the remaining 10 percent.

As a result, few scientists today believe that psychological problems directly cause infertility. But the pendulum may be swinging back, as specific reproductive actions of the brain are identified. The lower brain, or the hypothalamus, has been identified as the thrust behind the reproductive system, controlling the release of chemical signals that promote reproductive hormones from the pituitary gland and ultimately the ovaries. We know that 40 percent of infertility problems stem from ovulatory failure, which can theoretically be traced to the hypothalamus.

We also know that the hypothalamus is sensitive to psychological trauma, which can severely deplete the chemical signals that it sends to the pituitary gland. Certain drugs, particularly the psychiatric class of tranquilizers and mood modifiers, can override the hypothalamus and disturb the hormonal axis. Usually as soon as the drug is stopped the axis returns to normal. Illness and stress also can interfere with hormone production and thus temporarily stop ovulation.

The influence of the emotions and the brain on reproduction is a prime area of research. While psychological factors are not often considered a direct cause of infertility today, they are definitely considered a result. One of the most important discoveries to come out of modern fertility research is the recognition of an infertility stress syndrome. Infertility creates enormous emotional stress for both partners, and the stress increases as the couple goes through a workup and subsequent treatment. Stress can create problems in the marital relationship, and as well make existing problems worse. For these reasons, professional psychological evaluation is part of many fertility workups today.

Couples receive support to help them cope with stress, and scientists also gain some insight into stress factors that may be putting so much pressure on the couple that treatment cannot succeed. Fertility experts are cagey about linking emotional factors as a cause of infertility, but this new accumulated knowledge may ultimately help researchers learn why some couples, for unknown reasons, cannot conceive.

Any one—or more—of these factors may be involved when a woman finds herself unable to have a child. But an infertility problem may lie with a man as well. We know today that men, for a variety of reasons, have as high an incidence of infertility as do women.

INFERTILITY IN MEN

The commonest cause of infertility among men is a low sperm count, although it is rare for a man to have a complete absence of sperm in his semen. The causes of an abnormal sperm count are many and varied, and it's often impossible to distinguish one single disorder. Dozens of small problems, in themselves not especially destructive, can cluster together to reduce the sperm count. Because of the clustering of problems, treatment is often difficult and much less precise than it is in women, although the same fertility drugs are used to drive both systems. In men, the fertility specialist usually works with the overall system to improve general conditions in the hope that even a slightly elevated sperm count might be enough for pregnancy.

Fortunately, what some experts consider the most common cause of male infertility—a varicose vein of the testicle, called varicocele—is also the most successfully treated. Other causes include hormonal problems and chromosome abnormalities. Certain drugs and chemicals such as insecticides can also lower sperm counts. A man's fecundity also decreases somewhat with age, although not with the dramatic finality of female menopause.

Fertility problems may also be caused by infections, disease of the prostate gland or seminal vesicles, impotence, congenital defects in the penis, and several other factors, including blocked transport ducts or having had a hernia operation which may have damaged nearby reproductive organs.

For many men who have a low sperm count, however, there is no discernible cause.

Tests for Men

The foremost test of male fertility is the semen analysis, which is actually a series of tests carried out on a sample of masturbated seminal fluid. The semen analysis will reveal the number of sperm in the sample, as well as their shape and swimming ability. Other steps in a semen analysis examine the volume and quality of the seminal fluid.

Since every man produces some deformed sperm in his ejaculate, a man is considered fertile if, on analysis, his sperm are mainly healthy and exceed roughly fifty million per milliliter of semen, with more than half the sperm still swimming four hours after ejaculation.

A man may also have routine lab tests, and often blood tests to evaluate hormone levels. Another common test is the postcoital test, in which samples of mucus are removed from the woman's cervix within several hours after intercourse to see if healthy, moving sperm are present.

Today many fertility investigations include a psychological evaluation as well to determine the level of stress a couple may be suffering due to a prolonged struggle with infertility.

Treatment for Men
Infertility in men is much harder to treat than in women because it is often traced to more than one cause. Occasionally simple practical advice helps solve the problem. There is speculation that excess heat lowers sperm production. And jobs involving long hours of exposure to unusual heat may contribute to a lowered sperm count. When no other specific cause can be identified, infertile men are advised against tight underwear that holds the testicles close to the body.

A low sperm count can sometimes be improved by medical treatment with fertility drugs. A blockage in the ductal system can often be surgically corrected. About 40 percent of infertile men have varicocele, and surgery to tie off the varicose vein(s) is highly successful.

DOUBLE INFERTILITY

In about 30 percent of infertile couples, both partners have a problem. One thirty-six-year-old woman took fertility drugs for three years and underwent three microsurgical operations for tubal reconstruction in an effort to become pregnant—only to learn years later that her husband was infertile. It is not unusual for both partners to have one or more distinct fertility problems. It is also common, however, for both partners to be only slightly infertile, or "subfertile." A man may have a somewhat reduced sperm count; and, instead of regularly ovulating each month, a woman may ovulate every other month, or only three or four times a year. Matched with different, more fertile partners, each might produce children without noticeable difficulty. Together, however, they are infertile.

Jack had fathered two children with his first wife and saw no reason to undergo a fertility evaluation when his second wife, Vivian, was unable to conceive. She went through "every test in the book" over a period of five years and also took fertility drugs, without result. When Jack was finally tested his semen analysis showed a marginal sperm count. The solution for this couple was artificial insemination, which allows a greater number of sperm to reach the cervix and enter the uterus.

One unique, and highly controversial, infertility problem involves a so-called antibody reaction. For unexplained reasons some women seem to produce antibodies in their cervical mucus which kills or immobilizes sperm. In the same way, some men are believed to produce sperm-killing antibodies in their seminal fluid. These unusual, and speculative, causes of infertility are frustrating and difficult to successfully treat because so little is understood about them. In fact, andrologists do not even agree on the existence of the disorder.

Occasionally couples fail to achieve pregnancy simply because they don't have sex at the right time of the month, or because they use lubricants, such as Vaseline, which can immobilize sperm.

HOW TO GET HELP

Some fertility problems are easily resolved with help from your family physician or gynecologist. However, many problems require careful examination and treatment over a period of several months and sometimes years.

Getting help early can save time, money, and stress and ultimately increase the odds of a successful pregnancy. Even if you should fall into that small group in which no problem can be detected, consulting a specialist will reassure you that you have done everything you can to find an answer.

Fifteen years ago an international film star was told that she couldn't conceive because she had a "tipped" uterus. She received no further evaluation and, as a result, remained childless. If she had been evaluated by a competent specialist today, she would learn that there is no evidence that a so-called tipped uterus interferes with pregnancy; the fertility specialist would seek out the real cause of her infertility.

Here is one ironic statistic projected by a recent scientific study: in a large population of couples of all ages, about 20 percent will fail to achieve pregnancy within twelve months. If they all seek help from a fertility specialist, half of them will become pregnant in another six months—without any treatment. Therefore, if you haven't become pregnant in a specific length of time, it doesn't necessarily mean that you are infertile.

The next question is where to look for help. Exactly who—and what—is a fertility specialist? Someone who works with infertility, a subspecialty which crosses the boundaries of several different medical specialties: gynecology, urology, microsurgery, endocrinology, psychotherapy, and genetics. Ovulation, sperm production, conception, implantation of the fertilized egg in the uterus, and management of the early weeks of pregnancy all fall within the realm of the fertility expert.

Infertile couples may have to consult many different specialists merely to discover why they are infertile. Each specialist may have a different approach and recommend different treatment. Also mixed into the typical evaluation are laboratories and hospitals. The whole process may take several months.

According to leaders in the field, a medical team offers the best approach to fertility because it provides you with the greatest number of resources in the most organized manner. In a fertility team or clinic, one doctor acts as the team leader, working with a group of specialists. Ideally the team includes both male and female physicians and counselors, and treats both partners. You may not need the services of every specialist on the team, but they should consult together and review the overall picture.

The goal of a fertility workup is to provide precise answers within a given period of time. The physician(s) you choose should have a specific plan to recommend to you after your initial visit. In an orderly fashion the physician should outline for you what can be done and how long it will take for a diagnosis. He or she should also tell you the costs involved.

Several tests and examinations are required to provide a complete picture of the reproductive status of a couple. Even though the testing seems biased toward the female, full cooperation of both partners is crucial to a successful outcome. Even when only one person is worried, both partners should go together, even for the initial consultation. For both emotional and physical reasons, it's extremely important to consider infertility a shared concern. The timing and sequence of the tests ordered by the fertility specialist are important. The diagnostic tests themselves, derived from years of research by various investigators, are standard. But they should be performed in a specific sequence, and by expert technicians. The sequence may depend on a patient's age or previous medical history. A test performed at the wrong time is useless. Generally, nonsurgical tests are performed first.

For a woman, the investigation may include:

History and physical, diagnostic studies (temperature chart, postcoital test, blood tests for hormone levels, ultrasound, endometrial biopsy); surgical investigation to view the condition of the reproductive organs (hysteroscopy, laparoscopy, X-ray studies); chromosome analysis, if necessary.

For a man, the investigation may include:

History and physical, screening for varicocele, semen analysis. If indicated, other studies include hormone blood studies, testicular biopsy and X ray, chromosome analysis.

A workup is both costly and time-consuming. A full fertility workup that includes both partners can cost roughly twenty-five hundred to three thousand dollars, depending on where you live, and take two to six months to complete. In most cases, the longer the workup takes, the more it will cost. Costs also may rise if the tests are not coordinated, making repeat tests necessary. In the long run, the more efficiently the workup is planned, the less expensive it will be.

Every once in a while, even after a perfectly designed workup, a case is "unsolved." This does not mean that there will never be an answer; it means only that scientists have not yet learned everything there is to know about infertility.

In the last ten years scientists have been able to grasp significant facts about reproduction that had eluded them in the past. Fertility drugs have been developed that offer hope to thousands of couples; technology as well has come to grips with infertility. The marriage of the microscope and the surgical laser has made it possible to rebuild delicate reproductive structures within the pelvic cavity.

If a couple fails to achieve pregnancy with these remarkable new therapies, they may still get help from a wide array of new fertility enhancement techniques: artificial insemination, in vitro fertilization, embryo transfer, and others. The immediate future holds tremendous promise for infertile couples.

CHAPTER 18

FERTILITY ENHANCEMENT

DESPITE ADVANCES in medical and surgical treatment for infertility, today there are still many couples unable to have children. New fertility enhancement technologies may be the answer for some. Men who have a low or absent sperm count may benefit from artificial insemination. For women whose fallopian tubes are irreparably damaged or blocked by scar tissue, in vitro fertilization is now a possible alternative. Or a woman whose ovaries cannot produce healthy eggs might be able to have an embryo transfer. Or a surrogate mother may volunteer to carry a baby for a woman who has no uterus.

Before choosing fertility enhancement, couples need first to resolve their feelings about infertility. Not every person can accept the idea of having a child who inherits the genetic imprint of a stranger, or can face the sometimes arduous medical procedures that accompany many of these technologies. Nor should infertile couples feel they should seek out these treatments simply because they are available.

The authors of *The New Our Bodies Ourselves* raise some serious questions about the new technologies, questions that any couple thinking of using these advances will want to consider. They suggest that most of the money that goes into developing such supertechnologies would be better spent on preventive measures and basic health care services for all women. They also point out that fertility enhancement is more of a business venture than a health care imperative. Yet the publicity surrounding these technologies makes them seem imperative—that if a woman doesn't do everything in her power to fulfill her fertility potential she is letting down society. The authors also speak of the tendency of society as a whole to make women unable to bear children feel inadequate or unwomanly. In the course of researching infertility I spoke with many women who said they felt "diseased" and "abnormal" because they couldn't have children.

Wanting a baby and not being able to have one can be an intensely painful experience. And the extra pressure applied by society may encourage some women to go through time-consuming and expensive medical manipulations to have a child.

The other side of the picture is that at their best fertility enhancement technologies give couples who want children choices. And ultimately some of the work now being done in the reproductive sciences may help reduce hereditary diseases. The long-range potential of reproductive engineering is almost impossible to comprehend.

For the moment, one especially difficult aspect of all fertility enhancement techniques is their experimental status. With the exception of artificial insemination, these new techniques have a high failure rate. Couples should try to envision how they will feel if the process doesn't work, and they should decide how long they will keep trying if the technique fails the first time. These issues should be talked over before they agree to a new technique, because once a couple is in a program, stress abounds, making it difficult to clearly examine options. The best chance for success comes if both partners start out feeling stable, relaxed, and optimistic.

This chapter provides a condensed description of the fertility enhancement technologies currently available. With one exception, they are complicated, expensive, and have low success rates. However, couples desperately wanting a baby often feel that even some chance is a thousand times better than no chance at all.

ARTIFICIAL INSEMINATION

Artificial insemination is the least complicated and most successful alternative to natural conception. In artificial insemination from the husband (AIH) or from a donor (AID), a physician uses a small plastic tube to implant sperm directly into a woman's cervical canal.

The success rates for both forms of artificial insemination are generally equal to the natural pregnancy rates of fertile couples. AIH is used primarily when a husband has a low or abnormal sperm count. Collecting the sperm and implanting them at the cervical neck lets sperm bypass the harsh fluids of the female vagina. More sperm survive to enter the uterus and tubes, increasing the chance of fertilization. By special washing and separation techniques, AIH can also be used when a man's sperm are hampered by overly dense semen, when he produces only a few good quality sperm, or when the sperm clump together instead of swimming individually. Separation techniques can also be used in those rare instances of infertility when a man makes too many sperm.

AIH is simple and effective. (The technique can even be performed at home, although the success rate is somewhat reduced.) The procedure is performed just prior to or on the day of the woman's ovulation, anywhere from day ten to day sixteen of her menstrual cycle. Women who ovulate irregularly may need drug therapy to help develop and release the egg before they receive artificial insemination.

On the proper day the husband masturbates into a sterile glass jar, usually in a private room at the physician's office. Within about a half hour, the physician inserts a warm speculum into the woman's vagina and uses a syringe to push the semen into the neck of the cervix. Next, a silicone cup is inserted to hold the semen in place for several hours, until the sperm can penetrate the mucus and swim through the cervical canal into the uterus. There is no discomfort, and the woman removes the cup herself after about six hours.

Pregnancy rates with AIH correspond to those of natural pregnancy. A woman has about a 20 percent chance of pregnancy in the first month, a 50 to 70 percent chance by the third month, and an 80 percent chance by the end of six months.

Between one and three inseminations are performed in each menstrual cycle. Costs range from $150 to $450 for each month the technique is used; the higher cost is usual if a woman requires drug therapy.

Donor Sperm
When the male partner has little or no sperm, pregnancy can be achieved with donor sperm. A history of certain genetic disorders or

Rh incompatibilities also leads some couples to seek help from AID. Donor insemination may also be a choice when a couple has a long history of unexplained infertility. Currently, ten to twenty thousand children are born in the United States each year as a result of the AID procedure.

The disadvantage of the technique is that couples usually do not know the identity of the biological father, and little genetic screening is carried out on donors. So far the incidence of abnormalities with donor sperm does not appear to be greater than that in children born by natural insemination, but as the technique becomes more popular, this type of problem may arise more often. There have already been scattered reports of women artificially inseminated with donor sperm who contract the acquired immune deficiency syndrome (AIDS) virus.

If you are considering AID, ask your physician to take a medical history of the donor. Although the exact genetic mechanisms have not yet been uncovered, it is known that certain diseases—high blood pressure, heart disease, specific cancers—run in families. As the child grows into adulthood, an accurate family history, based on its biological parents, will assist any future medical evaluation and treatment. You might ask that the donor fill out a family medical work sheet, available through the local March of Dimes.

The technique for AID is the same as that for AIH, except that the donor sperm usually come from a sperm bank, which screens potential donors to some extent and collects their semen. The donor receives a nominal fee, generally about a hundred dollars. A record is usually kept of the donor's physical traits so that the physician can match some traits to those of the husband.

The physician selects the donor sperm, and the couple agrees to absolve the physician of responsibility for any abnormalities the child may have. If you are considering AID, try to find out the extent of screening carried out on donor sperm. Also ask how often the sperm bank allows one donor to provide sperm. The worry here is that in a small community the same person may donate sperm to more than one family; the offspring will be half siblings without recognizing the fact and there is a potential for intermarriage—an unlikely event, but a possibility.

Donor sperm today often come frozen, supplied by the sixteen major cryobanks in the United States. Typically, your physician orders frozen sperm from an anonymous donor in some other part of the country. He then defrosts the semen before insemination. Frozen sperm are usually more carefully screened for diseases or genetic defects. Further, the wide choice of donors lessens the possibility that two children fathered by the same donor might meet later in life and marry. Donor characteristics also can be more easily matched to the husband's physical characteristics—eye color, height, and so on.

The major problem is that defrosted sperm have a somewhat shorter life span than do fresh sperm, and insemination must be precisely matched with ovulation. The quality of the pregnancy does not appear to be affected by freezing of sperm, and the incidence of birth defects is no higher.

How Long to Keep Trying

Success rates for artificial insemination—either AIH or AID—vary widely. A recent medical journal reported that the average time for pregnancy was between 2.5 and 9.5 months. Theoretically, if you try long enough you will eventually become pregnant. Still, costs mount, and it's not easy to drop everything once or twice a month to see a physician for insemination. After six months of trying to achieve pregnancy, a couple should discuss the situation with their doctor. Poor timing may be at fault, in which case more sophisticated (and expensive) tests might be used to precisely pinpoint ovulation. Or the wife may have an undetected fertility problem which would require further testing and treatment.

Legal Snags

Artificial insemination donors are not informed about the use of their sperm, making it unlikely that a biological father will turn up years later and intrude into family relationships. Likewise, donors have never been held legally responsible for AID children. Most courts consider that the husband who consents to AID for his wife is the legal father of the child.

In general, the AID procedure involves these legal promises:

Before contributing semen each donor signs a form waiving all parental rights to any child conceived with his sperm. Before AID takes place, the husband promises in writing to accept the child as his own son or daughter. The agreement, usually signed by both husband and wife, spells out their understanding of the AID procedure; and the physician is not responsible for birth defects or other genetic abnormalities should they occur in the child.

This agreement is not necessarily valid in a court of law; nor does it take into account the multitude of legal issues that may arise later. For example, if a husband and wife divorce, who is responsible for the child? And there has been at least one instance where an AID-conceived child has wanted to know the identity of its biological father later in life.

Deciding for AID
Before any couple chooses the AID procedure, both partners should have a complete fertility workup. In many cases, allegedly infertile couples can have children with proper diagnosis and treatment. AID is not a first choice, then, but the result of careful evaluation.

Even when AID seems right for physical reasons, it may be wrong for emotional reasons. Many physicians suggest waiting at least six months after male infertility has been established to give the couple time to think things through. Partners should agree to AID only when both agree wholeheartedly. Large surveys have shown almost unanimous satisfaction among couples who have chosen the AID procedure, suggesting that when the circumstances are right it is a rewarding alternative to natural pregnancy.

IN VITRO FERTILIZATION (IVF)
Fertilization normally takes place in the woman's fallopian tubes when the newly released egg meets a sperm and begins to divide before implanting in the uterus. If the tubes are so damaged that the egg cannot make this journey, conception will not occur. The in vitro procedure creates a fertilization site outside the woman's body.

Seven years after the first "test-tube" baby was born in England, some seven hundred in vitro babies have been born worldwide. Many more pregnancies are in progress.

Today there are approximately 200 IVF clinics around the world, 121 of them in the United States. Many of these clinics, although their doors are open, have never had a successful pregnancy—that is, one that resulted in a live birth.

To achieve in vitro pregnancy couples must be prepared to invest much time and money, and the chances of success are low.

Who's a Candidate?

The main reason couples are accepted into in vitro programs is that the women have badly damaged fallopian tubes. However, today couples with a wide variety of fertility problems may be accepted for in vitro programs. Many clinics now accept women up to forty years of age, and older, though their chances of success are slim. Some clinics accept couples who have prolonged and unexplained infertility (five years or longer) or women who have persistent endometriosis. A few programs accept couples if the man has a low sperm count, although in these cases artificial insemination should be tried first, since it is far less expensive and less traumatic than in vitro fertilization.

In every case, regardless of other problems, at least one ovary must be normal and accessible. If a woman's ovaries are obscured by scar tissue or cysts she may first have to undergo microsurgery or laser surgery to free them. If she has difficulty ovulating, fertility drugs may be used to normalize her hormonal system. Above all, both partners must be free of infection of any kind.

Before a couple is accepted into a program, most clinics require a full workup from a fertility specialist. The medical records are then turned over to the in vitro clinic. Most clinics prefer to work through a referring physician, primarily because it ensures good follow-up care after the couple leaves the clinic.

The Technique

The basic steps of the in vitro procedure are these: remove an ovum from a woman, mix it with some sperm in a glass dish until one sperm penetrates the egg, then reimplant the fertilized egg into the woman's uterus. Success depends on precision timing, perfect matching of hormones, and luck.

The first sequence for in vitro fertilization is the same as natural conception: the growth and release of a mature egg. Timing of the sequence begins on the first day of a woman's menstrual cycle and ends with the transfer of the fertilized ovum into the uterus, usually on day fifteen. In vitro specialists usually want the woman to take fertility drugs for about five days to help the ovary produce several mature ova in a single month. (The evidence shows that the success rate improves when more than one fertilized egg is implanted in each cycle.)

As the eggs develop inside the ovary, the woman goes to the clinic daily for a series of ultrasound tests, which track their growth. Daily blood tests measure the rise of certain hormones in the blood. Together these tests will signal impending ovulation. The eggs need to be nearly mature, but not so mature that they leave the ovaries spontaneously.

Often another drug, human chorionic gonadotropin, is given to boost the eggs of the ovary at a precise time. Just before the eggs burst out of their follicles, usually on day thirteen of the cycle, the woman is taken to the operating room and given a general anesthetic. A member of the in vitro team inserts a laparoscope, a long slender telescope instrument, through her navel and gently suctions the eggs from the ovaries. Occasionally the eggs have failed to mature, and the woman must try again in a subsequent cycle. She usually recovers easily from the laparoscopy and remains in the hospital, waiting for the eggs to be fertilized and implanted in her uterus. The transfer to the uterus should take place within forty hours.

Once removed, the eggs are rushed to a highly specialized laboratory, where an expert in tissue culture bathes them in a special culture medium. The eggs are kept warm and allowed to mature fully while the sperm are prepared. Specialists agree that laboratory quality is the key to successful in vitro.

Each egg is then combined with a quantity of sperm in a glass dish and placed in an incubator. Fertilization usually takes place within twelve hours. The fused cell begins to divide, a sign that the embryo is developing normally.

Scientists have virtually mastered this initial sequence of the in vitro process. Up to this point, the procedure is successful 75 to 90 percent of the time.

The most difficult—and least successful—part of the in vitro process begins when the fertilized ovum (embryo) is transferred to the uterus.

When the fertilized ova have grown to either four or eight cells (researchers are still experimenting with the optimum time for transfer), they are drawn up into a catheter, along with a little neutral culture medium. The physician gently pushes the tip of the catheter through the woman's cervix and ejects the fluid column.

Following the transfer, a few days of bed rest are required to give the embryos time to implant. Overall, a fertilized egg implants only about 20 percent of the time in any one cycle. Of those that do implant one third spontaneously abort within the first twelve weeks, and another 10 to 15 percent abort later.

Because of the low odds of success most in vitro specialists implant more than one fertilized egg at a time, doubling or tripling the chances for a pregnancy. However, there is wide disagreement on just how many embryos should be used. Multiple implants may secrete too much estrogen, which affects the balance of the lining of the uterus and may endanger the embryos.

On the other hand, there have been fifty-six pairs of in vitro twins, eight sets of triplets and two sets of quadruplets. Experts suggest that the real danger of multiple implants is the stress and risk they place on the mother. Often women undergoing in vitro have had previous microsurgery and drug therapy. The strain of a multiple pregnancy can overstress the uterus and ultimately cause the miscarriage of all the fetuses in the womb.

Investigators are now trying to decide exactly what number of transfers improves the chances of pregnancy without drastically increasing the chances of multiple births. The medical issue is complicated by the moral implications. Some practitioners feel that all fertilized embryos should be implanted because each one is a living being. Since legal guidelines concerning the legal status of "extra embryos" have not been established, many American clinics transfer all embryos—as many as four or five at a time. However, the consensus of opinion expressed at a recent international medical seminar was that three to four eggs give the optimum results.

This issue may be resolved when in vitro researchers find a way to successfully identify the "best" eggs to fertilize. They reason that if only good quality eggs are fertilized they will have a better chance of implanting. Another solution may be the recent advance in embryo freezing, which means that all fertilized eggs would not have to be transferred at one time.

Risks of In Vitro
Even though in vitro fertilization takes place outside the body, a

woman faces several risks. These include the daily use of hormones, anesthesia during egg retrieval, general stress, and possible spontaneous abortion—which, of course, is the greatest risk to the embryo itself. Once a fetus comes to term, however, it doesn't seem to be at any greater risk of medical complications than a child conceived inside the body.

Success

Success rates vary widely among clinics and it's difficult to learn how successful a clinic has been because they report their statistics in several ways: by the number of successful fertilizations, by the number of successful transfers, by the number of pregnancies continuing beyond six to twelve weeks, and by the number of babies actually delivered. When you inquire, make sure the clinic identifies exactly which statistic it is giving you.

Overall, embryo transfer seems to succeed only about 20 percent of the time in any given cycle; within the first twelve weeks 33 percent of these transferred embryos spontaneously abort, and another 10 to 15 percent are lost to late abortion. This means that ultimately, a woman has only about a 10 percent chance that in vitro will result in a living baby in a given cycle.

The High Costs of In Vitro

Like all solutions to infertility, in vitro is expensive. These programs are not supported by state or federal funding, nor are they usually covered by health insurance.

Fees vary, but overall the technique costs from three to five thousand dollars for each cycle, including hospital fees. The first cycle, which usually includes fees for initial consultations and screening, is more expensive than subsequent cycles. To these medical fees you must add hidden costs—time off from work, travel, and hotel accommodations for two weeks or longer in each cycle.

The critical question is, how many cycles are needed to achieve pregnancy? And at what point should a couple stop trying? The story of the couple who has spent eighty thousand dollars so far—and is still trying—is not unusual. If the pregnancy takes and aborts several months later, the couple must decide whether they want to try again. Many clinics limit the number of attempts to three cycles; others say they will perform as many cycles as necessary to achieve pregnancy. In the future, the lengthy and complex in vitro process may be considerably streamlined, leading to a much shorter and less expensive process.

OTHER TECHNIQUES

Surrogate parenting is the most controversial of all fertility enhancement methods. In this case, the husband is fertile, but the wife is not. Another woman volunteers to become pregnant with the husband's sperm via artificial insemination and carry the baby to term. When the baby is born, the surrogate mother allows the couple to adopt the child. (Although the husband is the biological father of the child, in some states he is legally classified as a sperm donor, meaning that he has no legal right to or responsibility for the child. To guarantee a husband's rights, then, both husband and wife usually formally adopt the child of a surrogate mother.)

The biological basics of surrogate parenting are simple, but the emotional and practical aspects of the process are staggering. Looking at the legal and moral questions raised by dealing with life and birth and death in new ways has become the thorniest problem of our age. And nowhere are the issues more controversial than in surrogate parenting.

Like all fertility enhancement methods, surrogate parenting requires careful consideration of the deepest feelings of all three participants. Not every couple is emotionally suited to the procedure. Even when a husband and wife choose surrogate parenting, finding an appropriate surrogate and working out a contract is an involved process.

What are the couple's obligations should they separate or change their minds during the pregnancy? What if the baby is born with an unanticipated health problem? What if the surrogate changes her mind and decides she wants to keep the child?

What is the potential for financial gain by third parties? Is arranging for a surrogate, often a service performed by physicians and lawyers, the same thing as baby brokering? Although most surrogates request only a modest amount of money for a year of their lives—five thousand dollars is average—physicians' and lawyers' fees are sometimes exorbitant.

There are many pressures on both the couple and the surrogate.

Social and religious strictures can be stressful for all three parties. The surrogate goes through the additional stress of carrying a child for nine months, then may be faced with sadness and guilt when the time comes to give the child up for adoption.

The only large study examining the motivation of surrogates found that while money was one motivation they had in common, it was by no means the dominant reason that they volunteered. Many of the 173 women interviewed said that they wanted to help a deserving couple; others said they could enjoy the experience of pregnancy without the responsibility of caring for the child.

The legal status of surrogate parenting is in limbo. There is no state or federal legislation in place that makes it legal or illegal. The few states that have any laws on the subject mainly prohibit payment for such an act, not necessarily the act itself.

The couple and the surrogate sign a contract, a standard part of the surrogate procedure. The contract spells out the costs, risks, and responsibilities of each person. Even though these contracts are devised with the help of a lawyer, they are not necessarily legally valid. The major risk, from the viewpoint of the couple, is that the surrogate mother will decide to keep the baby after giving birth. If the surrogate mother changes her mind at any time, even years in the future, the couple may have no legal recourse.

Some of the issues were highlighted in one well-publicized case. A severely retarded baby was born to a surrogate mother, and the couple who contracted for the child refused to accept it. Their reason? Medical tests proved that even though the surrogate was inseminated with the husband's sperm, he was not the father of the child.

At the time of the contract, the surrogate was separated from her own husband. A few days before the artificial insemination the surrogate had sexual intercourse with her estranged husband, whose family had a history of birth defects. The surrogate and her husband were the biological parents of the child.

The result was that every party involved in the contract, including the physician, who supposedly had not advised the surrogate against intercourse before artificial insemination, filed and counterfiled a lawsuit, and the entanglement still has not been resolved.

Even with the potential for legal problems, however, many couples proceed with the arrangement and take the chance that the surrogate they choose will honor the agreement. Attorney Lori B. Andrews has elaborated on many of the legal complexities of surrogate parenting in her book *New Conceptions*, which is recommended for anyone contemplating fertility enhancement techniques.

Embryo Transfer

In January of 1984 at the Harbor-University of California at Los Angeles Medical Center, a woman gave birth to a baby that had been conceived in the body of another woman. Embryo transfer, devised by Dr. John E. Buster, may be the solution for couples who are infertile because the woman's ovaries cannot produce healthy eggs. As long as she has a healthy uterus, she can nurture a fetus. The infant carries the genes of the woman's husband and the donor woman.

Here's how embryo transfer works. A female donor volunteers to be inseminated with the husband's sperm. If she conceives, the doctors flush the embryo from her uterus five to six days later and implant it into the uterus of the wife. Embryo transfer is easier than in vitro because it requires no surgery to retrieve the ova. Fertilization occurs in the natural fertilization site, the fallopian tubes. The key to the transfer process is the precise matching of menstrual cycles of the two women.

There are some serious risks:

The embryo may not be washed out with the fluid, leaving the donor pregnant; the embryo may be flushed back into the tube, leaving the donor with an ectopic pregnancy; and the donor risks ectopic pregnancy, and also pelvic infection.

Because so few embryo transfers have been attempted in humans, it's difficult to predict the potential success rate if the technique is perfected. However, the technique is known to have a high success rate in animal breeding.

The Future

Researchers foresee a time when egg banks will be as popular as sperm banks. With egg banks, donor eggs can be fertilized in vitro and the embryos frozen. In that manner, embryos can be transferred to the uterus of an infertile woman at the appropriate time.

The same principle of embryo transfer could be used in reverse: a woman who has a defective uterus could have her egg fertilized with her husband's sperm in vitro and then implanted in another woman, who becomes the surrogate. This combination of in vitro and surrogate could also be used by women who cannot carry a child because of a medical condition unrelated to fertility, such as high blood pressure.

By the year 2000, enthusiasts for embryo transfer say it may be possible to flush the embryos from every pregnant woman as part of routine prenatal care, test it for genetic defects and then, if the embryo is perfect, return that embryo to the woman's womb.

Although scientists and infertile couples around the world are enthusiastic about these medical advances, the future of fertility enhancement is closely tied to the viewpoints of many different kinds of people, including religious leaders, philosophers, physicians, lawyers, and politicians. Women's groups also are becoming more outspoken in questioning the validity of the high costs charged to infertile couples for these advances. In the future the ability of an infertile couple to have children may be limited not by medical technology but by decisions made by judges in the courtrooms of America.

In this section we have looked at some of the high-risk categories for pregnancy today: hereditary defects, preexisting diseases, chronic miscarriage, advanced age, and infertility. Only twenty years ago women and men who fell into any of these categories could often expect to give up their hopes for having a family. Today medical science has made enormous strides in every one of these groups, and it is only the beginning. Having children with good planning and preparation in advance of conception, and quality prenatal care during pregnancy, can be healthy and safe for most people in every one of these high-risk groups.

PART FOUR

READY FOR PREGNANCY

CHAPTER 19

NEW TRENDS IN
MATERNITY CARE

PREGNANCY AND CHILDBIRTH are universal events for which scientists continually seek newer and better technology. Newspapers and magazines and television programs daily report the development of some remarkable new invention or diagnostic procedure. Readers and listeners are bombarded with technical information and conflicting viewpoints about methods of delivery. For anyone contemplating parenthood, such a barrage of data can be confusing and often overwhelming.

Again, your choices are broad, and it takes information and consideration to decide what kind of obstetrical care is best for you. It's also important to begin prenatal care as soon as your pregnancy is confirmed, which means that you won't have much time for shopping around after you become pregnant. It's much more practical, and ultimately more rewarding, to think through your options before pregnancy.

Standards of maternity care are sensitive to even minor fluctuations in social trends. In recent years women have created a substantial backlash against the impersonalized, technical methods of delivery which, in the name of safety and progress, seemed to serve the convenience of the doctors and hospital staff more than the needs of the parents.

Many women and some physicians today view pregnancy as a healthy condition and see no reason for labor and childbirth to take place in a sterile, mechanical hospital environment. They believe that babies and mothers do best when childbirth is accompanied by as little medical interference as possible.

Many obstetricians, on the other hand, argue that when things go wrong during delivery they go wrong suddenly and often without warning. Having the latest and best technology available at a moment's notice is the best way to ensure the safety of mother and baby.

An American sort of compromise has evolved, in which some hospitals, still sporting their numerous technological advantages, have tried to become more homelike for mothers and babies. Many hospitals now have birth rooms, flexible visiting hours, and rooming in for the newborn. This personalized approach is complemented by technological advances that make childbirth today safe even for many complicated pregnancies.

These new trends in maternity care, which include childbirth classes for both partners and the father's participation in labor and delivery, are called family-centered.

Not every obstetrician and hospital today take a family-centered approach. It is still up to parents to search for an obstetrician and hospital that meet their own personal preferences. Instead of hospitals, some couples choose to have their babies at home or in a birthing center, but although these options are increasing neither trend is widespread at this time.

CHOOSING AN OBSTETRICIAN

A good obstetrician can be hard to find these days. Due to rising costs of malpractice insurance associated with obstetrics many physicians are abandoning this specialty in favor of less demanding, less potentially risky fields. Nurse-midwives are also faced with similar escalating insurance costs that are forcing many out of practice. The search is complicated by the fact that not only do you want to find competent prenatal care, you want to find someone you *like*—someone with whom you're glad to share this most important experience of your life.

This makes the search for obstetrical care a major concern, and one that you need to spend time on. Ideally your search should begin before conception so that prenatal care can begin as soon as you become pregnant. When you have a baby in America today you have several different types of maternity care to choose from.

An Obstetrician in Private Practice

You can start by asking your family doctor and close friends for a recommendation. Another way is to ask a resident in obstetrics and gynecology or an obstetrical nurse at a local hospital for the name of a competent obstetrician. If he or she is reluctant to recommend one particular doctor, ask for a list of two or three names. A childbirth education group or a branch of the La Leche League, a worldwide organization that offers new mothers instruction for successful breast-feeding, can provide you with names of obstetricians in your area.

The doctor you choose may be a general practitioner, a family doctor, a gynecologist, or an obstetrician. Although many excellent general practitioners practice obstetrics, they may not have the experience to handle a high-risk obstetrical case, so your age and medical history may influence your choice.

Many obstetricians are board-certified by the American Board of Obstetrics and Gynecology or "board eligible," meaning that a physician has met all the requirements but has not yet passed the board examinations. Board certification means that obstetricians have spent four to five years in resident's training after they have received their initial medical degrees, and that they have passed several difficult examinations.

Another indication of competence is if the doctor is affiliated with a hospital with an approved residency program for obstetrics or one attached to a medical school. The *Directory of Medical Specialists* and the *American Medical Directory*, available at public libraries, are both excellent source books that list qualifications and affiliations of specialists.

When it comes to choosing a doctor, gender may be important to you. At this time, only a small percentage of obstetricians in the United States are women. However, women make up a much larger percentage of the obstetrical residents currently training in university teaching centers, which suggests that in the future there will be many more women obstetricians.

Your purpose at this point is to accumulate the names of several obstetricians. Don't hesitate to shop around; make an appointment to meet with more than one doctor or go to more than one clinic before making your decision. You will probably have to pay for the consultations, but in the long run making a good choice at first can save you the later unhappiness.

Arrange an initial meeting with the doctor, preferably with your husband or partner present. Before meeting the physician, make a list of questions you want to ask.

When you meet with a doctor, remember that credentials are not everything. Nor are the most expensive physicians necessarily the most highly qualified.

Certainly, the doctor you choose should instill confidence and offer superior care and technical expertise. But he or she should also have time to answer your questions and to discuss various kinds of labor and delivery methods. He or she will want to know how you are feeling and be genuinely concerned for your welfare. The most important thing is to find a physician who is competent and caring, someone you can trust.

In addition to the individual physician in private practice, other kinds of obstetrical care are available, each with its own advantages. You will want to consider each in the context of your own preferences and circumstances.

Group Practice
Many obstetricians today ease the round-the-clock demands of obstetrics by joining in group practice. A group may be anything from two doctors to ten.

If you choose a group practice, try to get to know every doctor in the group, even if just one obstetrician follows you through your pregnancy. There is always the possibility that a different member of the group will be with you at the time of delivery.

If you feel uncomfortable with one member of the group, request that another doctor attend your labor and delivery, even if your nonrapport doctor is on call. If this can't be promised, it might be worth it to look further. Each birth is a once-in-a-lifetime experience for a couple, and the attending physician is an integral part of that experience.

Hospital Clinics
Some couples opt for maternity care in a hospital clinic staffed by resident obstetricians, obstetrical nurses, and often nurse-midwives. You visit the clinic just as you would a private obstetrician, begin-

ning with prenatal checkups straight through delivery. Clinics also offer childbirth preparation classes.

One advantage is that hospital maternity clinics also have available many different kinds of specialists. Another is that clinic costs are generally lower than private care, but vary considerably. Some clinics, for example, have a sliding pay scale, so cost will depend on your income.

Hospital Midwife Programs

One new trend in maternity care offered by a few hospital clinics is the presence of nurse-midwives. A nurse-midwife is qualified to deliver babies and remains with the mother throughout labor to provide psychological as well as medical support. A nurse-midwife specializes in low-risk pregnancies. In some hospitals an obstetrician is always present at the birth, in others an obstetrician is available as backup in case of complications.

A midwife is a graduate registered nurse who has completed a one- to two-year course in nurse-midwifery. She has also passed the national certification exam given by the American College of Nurse-Midwives and uses the initials G.N.M. after her name.

Birthing Centers

Another relatively new phenomenon on the American scene is a small out-of-hospital facility called a birthing center. Only healthy, young, low-risk mothers are accepted for care at a birthing center, which is usually staffed by midwives, with obstetricians on call for backup.

The advantage is that centers have none of the institutionalized atmosphere of a hospital. For example, one in New York is located in a town house on a quiet, beautiful tree-lined street. Most centers offer full maternity care, including childbirth classes and delivery, and the costs are generally lower than those of hospital delivery. You may be unable to find a birthing center near you, however, because there are only 125 such facilities nationwide.

A list of birthing centers can be found in the yellow pages of your telephone book; on request the American College of Nurse-Midwives (1522 K Street NW, Washington, D.C. 20005) will provide you with a list of nurse-midwife services in your area.

QUESTIONS TO ASK

Prospective parents today have a lot to say about the manner in which they would like to have their baby delivered, particularly if the pregnancy is low-risk. Different approaches to labor and delivery appeal to different people.

Read current magazine articles and other publications about new delivery methods and talk them over with friends who have recently had babies. You might also want to visit a local hospital with a well-known obstetrical unit to learn how deliveries are being handled there.

Even if you're not sure what approach you would like, discuss various possibilities with your obstetrician or midwife on your first prenatal visit. Show that you have given the matter thought, but at the same time keep an open mind and listen to what the doctor has to say.

When you and your physician have agreed (and you may have to alter your choice of delivery method if circumstances change after you go into labor), review your plan with the hospital or birthing center well in advance of delivery.

If the doctor or hospital staff will not agree to your requests, or if you feel uncomfortable with the place or person you have chosen, consider interviewing another obstetrician and/or hospital.

CHOOSING A HOSPITAL

Hospitals also need to be selected ahead of time, particularly if you live in a metropolitan area with many facilities to choose from. The trend for many hospitals today is family-centered maternity care.

Hospitals that take this approach usually encourage your partner or a friend to participate in labor and delivery and allow other family members unrestricted visiting hours. Some hospitals also provide nurse-midwives to stay with you from the beginning of labor all the way through delivery. A few family-centered hospitals have established birthing rooms, in which delivery as well as labor takes place. The birthing room usually looks like a living room or bedroom. In case complications arise, the mother can quickly be wheeled to the nearby delivery room and the infant taken to a neonatal unit for specialized care. If you choose a hospital because it has a birthing room, however, remember that there is no guarantee that the room will be free when you're ready to give birth.

The best way to evaluate a hospital is to take a tour of the maternity unit. The hospital you choose should be willing to give you such a tour, including labor and delivery rooms. Nurses should freely describe visiting hours and all other regulations that would affect your stay.

The approach of the hospital may be important enough to you that you might consider choosing the hospital first, then finding an obstetrician who is affiliated with it.

No matter what kind of hospital you choose, you will want to know if the hospital is equipped to handle an emergency should one arise. If you know in advance that yours is a high-risk pregnancy you will want to choose a hospital known for its superior technology and neonatal unit.

You will also want to know if the hospital will allow your pediatrician to come in to examine your baby right after it is born. Most important is early and accurate diagnosis of any difficulties, so that the baby can either be treated or moved for treatment immediately. Should it become necessary for the baby to be transferred to another hospital for special care, find out how far away the transfer unit is and if you will be moved with your child.

PREPARED CHILDBIRTH CLASSES

In the second or third trimester of pregnancy, many couples attend prepared childbirth classes together. In these classes you will learn what to expect in each stage of labor and practice relaxation and breathing techniques for each one.

The concept of prepared childbirth classes is that a couple should become familiar with the sequence of events of normal labor. The mother will learn how she can help herself during the various phases and her partner will learn how to help her.

Most incorporate various breathing and relaxation techniques into a generalized program based on the Lamaze method. Some classes offer a slightly different approach, such as the Bradley method. A good class is practical as well as theoretical. The teacher should give basic information about the physiological changes of pregnancy, explain about vaginal and cesarean deliveries, anesthesia, and pain relief, and include open discussions about various childbirth and hospital techniques.

Toward the end of your course you will be told what to expect if you need an episiotomy or a cesarean section and what your doctor will do if something goes wrong during labor or delivery. Ideally, your class will include instructions on breast-feeding and bottle-feeding as well as other postnatal advice.

At the very least, prenatal classes help you know what to expect when labor begins. No matter when you are having your baby, or what kind of prenatal care you have chosen, you will want to learn about the physiology of pregnancy and labor, as well as the different ways of coping with labor and birth.

Even if this is not your first pregnancy, it's wise to remind yourself about the different ways of relaxing and breathing during labor. Too you will want to know about any changes in obstetric procedures since your last baby was born.

Prepared childbirth classes give you the opportunity to meet other couples with whom you can discuss your anxieties, plans, and hopes. Many couples meet other couples in childbirth classes who become lifelong friends.

Prepared childbirth classes have become the mainstay of good maternity care in the United States, but they are still a relatively new idea, based on the principle that fear creates physical tension, which in turn makes pain worse. This was the conclusion of an English physician, Dr. Grantly Dick-Read, who developed the earliest theories of natural childbirth in the 1920s.

Dick-Read observed hundreds of women in labor and noted that women who had not acquired a fear of labor did not experience the pain normally associated with childbirth. Frightened women appeared to suffer more. He concluded that labor was natural and inherently joyful because of its positive result.

Dick-Read's notion was that by simple instruction and a gentle approach to labor fear could be eliminated. And if fear was eliminated or reduced, labor would be easier. Dick-Read did not claim that childbirth was pain-free or that medication did not have a place in complicated labor.

Dick-Read's approach became popular in Britain and the United States, but in the 1950s it was gradually superseded by the Lamaze method, which more actively involves a woman in her labor and delivery.

Dr. Fernand Lamaze was a French physician who based his technique on the Pavlovian principle of conditioned response. Untrained, the whole body instinctively tenses during a contraction. With practice a woman can learn to relax the rest of her body when a labor contraction occurs. This deliberate relaxing minimizes tension throughout the body, making subsequent contractions less painful. The Lamaze method also emphasizes the role of a trained labor coach.

Today, Dick-Read's basic premise, the fear-tension-pain connection, is still acknowledged in most prepared childbirth courses. The Lamaze method, however, which emphasizes the active participation of the mother and her partner in a sequence of trained responses, forms the basis of most classes.

More recently the Bradley method, which emphasizes the intimate participation of the husband in all phases of the pregnancy and birth, has become popular. Over an extensive six-month course a pregnant woman and her partner are taught to recognize any sign of tension in her body and how to eliminate it by touch and massage techniques.

All the newer prepared childbirth methods have some common denominators based on the notion that birth is often a tough and demanding process. All classes stress physical training, muscle relaxation, and learning specialized breathing techniques for the different phases of labor.

The goal is that the mother will be able to respond to contractions with relaxation and breathing techniques which release tension, facilitate labor, and require so much concentration that she is distracted from much of the discomfort. Prepared childbirth helps eliminate fear. The emphasis is on being awake and aware during this significant life experience.

What It Isn't

Contrary to widely held misconceptions, prepared childbirth is not necessarily "painless" childbirth, nor are you expected to go through labor and delivery without medication or medical help. The ability to cope with pain varies considerably from person to person, as does the intensity and duration of pain itself. In most classes various medications are fully described and are regarded as tools to aid labor. If during the course of labor you decide that the pain is more than you can tolerate, you are expected to ask for medication. Prepared childbirth training does help you reduce tension and thus decrease pain; psychological techniques rarely abolish pain completely and are not equally effective for everyone. The effect of two or more techniques used together, however, appears to be cumulative. Most teachers of prepared childbirth classes advise that no matter how much you want to remain in control, you should never be ashamed to ask for or to accept analgesics or anesthesia at some stage of labor and delivery. Excessive anxiety and stress in labor and delivery could be worse than the possible side effects of medication.

Reserving a Spot

You can start looking into various childbirth classes at any time, but make sure to make your choice and reserve a place by your twelfth week of pregnancy. You should start classes by the time you are twenty-eight to thirty-two weeks pregnant.

Prepared childbirth classes may be run by a hospital, a community organization, such as the Y, or by individual instructors. Your doctor can probably recommend a class to you.

Prepared childbirth classes vary somewhat from class to class. Almost all classes encourage the participation of your partner or a friend. Classes are usually limited to ten couples and are often smaller. Most two-hour classes meet once a week for six weeks. Sometimes, additional classes are offered during the early months of pregnancy to deal with physical changes and emotional adjustments.

If you are not sure which class to choose, ask the teacher if you can sit in on a class to get an idea of what it is like. Teachers who are concerned about the well-being of new parents will usually agree.

A reputable teacher need not be a registered nurse, but she should provide details about her qualifications and experience. The teacher should guide discussions, rather than simply lecture. Every prepared childbirth class should be a shared experience, with everyone having a chance to participate. Ideally, the teacher will also offer an all-around, unbiased insight into childbirth and parenthood.

Your Labor Partner

A basic aspect of prepared childbirth classes is developing a close working relationship with your partner. Your partner will comfort and support you during labor. He or she will keep you from being alone or afraid and will help boost your morale if labor becomes trying. The exercises you learn together will be the tools you both use to help sustain you during labor and delivery.

If the baby's father is not your partner, you should choose a labor companion early in pregnancy. You may want to ask your mother or sister or a close friend to be your companion. Whoever you choose should be free to attend the childbirth classes with you and be willing to learn the breathing techniques. He or she should also be free to be with you on a moment's notice as the time for labor approaches.

Despite all your plans and the good intentions of your partner there is always a possibility that something will happen at the last minute to prevent your labor partner from being with you. You should always be prepared for this possibility and know that should such circumstances prevail you will be able to manage alone.

Of all the trends creeping into the established medical conventions prepared childbirth classes are perhaps the most significant and destined to be the most long-lasting. They are among the important steps in a nationwide trend to educate everyone in medicine and health care, giving each person more control over his or her life, and letting each make better choices. Like every aspect of pregnancy and childbirth the wide variety of available courses means that you need time to explore ahead of time so that when you become pregnant you will be able to be reserved in the class of your choice.

All of our discussion so far has been devoted to everything you can do beforehand to prepare yourself for pregnancy. The final chapter of *The Pre-Pregnancy Planner* takes you into those early days after you have become pregnant: what you can expect to happen and the adjustments you can anticipate making in your life over the next three months.

CHAPTER 20

THE FIRST WEEKS
OF PREGNANCY

WHEN YOU STOP USING a contraceptive you may become pregnant almost immediately. Or you may not become pregnant for several months. The anticipation of conception can be exciting, and sometimes nerve-racking.

EARLY SYMPTOMS OF PREGNANCY

The first symptoms of pregnancy may not appear until several weeks after you conceive. A missed period may be the first sign, but it is by no means an accurate barometer. As has been said, there are other causes of a missed period. Some women miss a period when they stop taking the pill. Exercise and dieting may also cause you to miss a period. So can emotional stress and illness. Even worry about becoming pregnant or extreme eagerness to have a baby can blunt menstruation.

Conversely, it is possible to be pregnant and still have menstrual bleeding. A partially suppressed period, caused by insufficient progesterone, may occur once or twice but seldom continues throughout pregnancy.

Some women feel light-headed and experience pregnancy sickness soon after the first missed period. Breasts may feel heavy and full. During the first twelve weeks of pregnancy some women have to urinate frequently, probably due to hormonal changes affecting kidney function, or the enlarging uterus pressing slightly on the bladder.

Other early symptoms of pregnancy are a heavy feeling in the lower abdomen and tiredness. As soon as you even suspect you are pregnant, you should have a pregnancy test so that if it is positive you can begin early prenatal care.

TESTING FOR PREGNANCY

The most commonly used pregnancy tests detect pregnancy by measuring the hormone HCG in a woman's blood or urine one to two weeks after a missed period. HCG is produced by the embryo and is normally not present unless a woman is pregnant.

Urine tests are about 98 percent accurate, but false results sometimes occur if the test is done too soon, or if the sample is not properly handled.

Today you can have your family doctor or a clinic perform your pregnancy test, or you can do it yourself using a home kit. The time it takes to get the result of the test can range from a few hours, if it is done on the premises, to a few days if the urine is sent to a laboratory. Home kits give the result in one or two hours.

Home tests vary slightly in method, but they all work on the principle of adding chemicals to urine in a test tube, leaving it undisturbed for a specified time, then reading the result. Home kits can be used from one to five days after a period should have begun.

All pregnancy tests should be done on a sample of the first urine you pass in the morning when the concentration of HCG is at its peak. Before collecting the sample you should not have anything to drink, nor should you have urinated during the night. You collect the urine in a clean jar, free of any trace of soap or detergent, then close the lid tightly and store the jar until the sample is tested.

New Tests

A new range of highly sensitive laboratory tests for pregnancy are becoming available. Two of the new tests work by detecting HCG in the blood, with a greater sensitivity that allows accuracy about a week after *conception* and also gives an idea of how long the woman has been pregnant. A third test, which uses monoclonal antibodies to detect pregnancy about two weeks after conception, can be done in the physician's office.

YOUR FIRST PRENATAL VISIT

As soon as you discover you are pregnant, you should have your first prenatal checkup. The number of prenatal checks you have through pregnancy depends largely on your medical history. Most women see their obstetricians once a month until the twenty-eighth week of pregnancy. As they enter the last trimester, they see their doctors every other week until week thirty-six, then every week until labor begins.

The first prenatal visit involves a complete medical workup, beginning with a thorough medical history that includes family background and history of previous pregnancies. If you have had a pre-pregnancy checkup, this information may already be recorded. The standard prenatal examination includes taking your blood pressure, an internal vaginal examination, breast exam, blood tests, and urinalysis.

Now is the time to talk over anything that worries you. If you tend to forget your questions the minute you walk into a doctor's office, write them down beforehand and bring them along.

DATING THE BIRTH

On your first prenatal visit your obstetrician will work out the date the baby is due to arrive. The average period of gestation is 266 days —or thirty-eight weeks—from the date of conception. However, since the exact time of conception is impossible to determine, doctors count 280 days, or forty weeks, from the first day of your last period. (This assumes that you have a regular twenty-eight-day menstrual cycle and that ovulation took place on day fourteen.)

Obviously every woman's menstrual cycle does not conform to a twenty-eight-day pattern and, even if it did, this method is open to slight inaccuracies. In addition, the duration of an individual pregnancy may vary considerably from the average and still be normal. It isn't surprising, therefore, that as many as 40 percent of all labors start more than seven days before or after the estimated date of delivery.

THE FETUS IN THE FIRST TWELVE WEEKS

A baby begins life as a single cell. Immediately after the chromosomes of the sperm and egg come together in the upper reaches of one fallopian tube, the new fused cell divides within its containing bubble and begins to move down the fallopian tube toward the uterus. With each division, the new cells, called blastomeres, become smaller.

About sixty hours after ovulation, the new cell cluster contains between twelve and sixteen blastomeres, and it sails from the narrow tunnel of the fallopian tube into the relatively huge cavern of the uterus.

The whole cluster is no bigger than the original egg. On entering the uterus, however, the cluster—now called a blastocyst—begins a new phase of development with its physical attachment to the endometrial lining of the uterus.

The blastocyst is a tiny hollow sphere of cells bulging at one end. The bulge is the raw material from which the embryo will grow. The sphere wall implants on the back wall of the uterus and becomes the connecting link between the embryo and the mother.

Sometimes a blastocyst implants in other places—usually with serious consequences. If the blastocyst implants near the cervical end of the uterus, heavy bleeding in the last stages of pregnancy may occur, as well as other complications during delivery.

Other wrongly targeted implantations may lead to ectopic pregnancies, which miscarry with heavy bleeding early in pregnancy.

By about day nine or ten, the blastocyst buries itself in the wall of the uterus and disappears, its position marked only by a small clot of blood remaining on the surface. In the next few weeks the foundations of the baby's body are laid and the placenta, the complex structure that will sustain the baby's growth, begins to form.

The bulge, called an embryoblast, divides into two layers. One layer gives rise to the outer surface—the skin and hair—then folds inward to make the nervous system. The second layer creates the inner surface of the body—the alimentary tract, the liver, and the lungs.

During the third week of development, a third cell layer fills in between the two original layers and ultimately builds such vital body systems as the muscles and blood. By about day twenty-one the embryo has changed from a sheet of undistinguished cells into a distinct head and tail fold.

Other changes have occurred around the bulging embryo. The wall surrounding the embryo has thickened considerably; finger-shaped processes called villi grow out of the wall and poke into the surrounding tissue of uterine lining.

A pocket of fluid now separates the embryo from its surrounding wall, and a connecting stalk develops between the two.

The fourth to eighth weeks of human development are called the embryonic period, dominated by dramatic changes in the nervous system and blood supply. It is in these very early days that the embryo is especially vulnerable to environmental damage. Early sets of primitive cells align themselves in ladderlike progressions that eventually change into cartilage, bones, and muscles.

During the fourth or fifth week, a minute primitive heart begins to pump newly formed blood cells around the pea-sized embryo. By the sixth week the circulatory system becomes established and the heart is strongly beating.

The embryo's head is large in proportion to the rest of its body, but the eyes and nostrils, which were at the side of the head, have now moved to the front. The eyes are covered by skin that will form the eyelids, and they will remain closed until week twenty-five or twenty-six. The inner ear is rapidly growing, but the external ear has not yet formed.

The embryo's limbs are growing and by week seven its hands and feet have formed. By the end of week eight the baby's embryonic period is complete, and it now enters the fetal period and is called a fetus, meaning offspring.

By twelve weeks after conception, the limbs and internal organs of the fetus are fully formed, although they are not sufficiently developed for it to survive independently. The external sex organs are now developed enough for the baby's sex to be determined by ultrasound inspection.

The amniotic sac which surrounds the fetus contains about twelve ounces of fluid and the three-inch fetus has plenty of room to move about, although the mother cannot feel it move yet. For the remainder of the pregnancy the baby will grow and mature.

YOUR CHANGING DIET

As the baby grows and develops, your need for protein, minerals, and other nutrients increases. You need nearly twice as much protein, calcium, and vitamin C as usual. Certain B vitamins and folic acid are also much more important during pregnancy. Iron intake is vital.

For the most part, however, the idea is to continue to follow a well-balanced diet but increase the number or amount of servings. The extra calories you consume should be packed with protein, calcium, vitamins, and other nutrients. Three Cokes, for example, equal three hundred calories, but those calories won't help you or your baby.

Vitamin Supplements

Many obstetricians today believe that it is not absolutely essential for pregnant women to take vitamin and mineral supplements, provided they are eating a well-balanced diet. Nevertheless, certain prenatal supplements are often recommended, particularly folic acid. But supplements should be taken only on the advice of your obstetrician.

Too Many Vitamins

Certain vitamins are known to cause serious problems if taken in excess. Large doses of vitamin A, vitamin D, and zinc can be poisonous to your unborn baby. These vitamins should be consumed only in natural foods, which makes it virtually impossible to overdose. The popular vitamin C supplement, which many people take today, can also be a problem for your baby. When a fetus receives large quantities of vitamin C in utero it may suffer a vitamin deficiency after birth, when it no longer receives an excess supply. If you feel you need supplementary vitamin C, consult your obstetrician to learn safe levels.

PREGNANCY SICKNESS

A common problem of early pregnancy is pregnancy sickness. Approximately 70 percent of pregnant women experience some form of sickness, ranging from mild nausea in the morning to all-day nausea and frequent vomiting. (The term "morning sickness" is a misnomer because most pregnant women experience sickness off and on all day long.) Pregnancy sickness does not threaten the life of the mother or baby, but for a few women it can be especially miserable. Pregnancy sickness, like other changes of pregnancy, is caused by a disturbance in the normal working systems of the body. A high level of HCG usually coincides with sickness, suggesting that this pregnancy hormone is the culprit. Other hormones also may be involved. Another important factor may be a woman's diet, both before and in the early weeks of pregnancy. One study suggests that women whose diets are high in protein and low in carbohydrates and vitamin B_6 may have more trouble with sickness. Older women also seem to suffer from more severe sickness. And emotional stress at any age seems to make pregnancy sickness worse.

Feeling Better
You can't really cure pregnancy sickness, but several things will help minimize illness. Diet, mild exercise, and rest are the main ingredients.

A well-balanced diet with the emphasis on unrefined carbohydrates, such as whole wheat bread and pasta, whole grain cereals, wheat germ, bananas, and other fresh fruit, usually helps reduce pregnancy sickness, possibly because these foods are high in vitamin B_6. (Foods rich in fat—fried foods and red meat—tend to make nausea worse.)

If you cannot face the "good" foods, eat whatever you can tolerate even if you just nibble. As far as holding down nausea goes, you will feel better when you eat. Fasting tends to make things worse. So, eat the foods you like and drink plenty of fluids so you don't become dehydrated.

If you were well nourished before you became pregnant, your body will sustain you now. You will have time to make up for any deficiencies after the pregnancy sickness passes and you resume a nutritious eating pattern.

Tips
Try eating several small meals throughout the day, especially in the morning, instead of three larger ones. If you can eat a large meal, have it in the middle of the day rather than in the evening.

A snack before going to bed, even if you don't feel like it, will help soothe morning nausea. Your mother's advice to keep a box of dry crackers next to your bed and nibble on one when you wake up in the morning actually works—it helps settle your stomach.
Drinking plenty of fluids will help neutralize the acids in your stomach. Chewing on small pieces of ice helps some women. Carry caramels or hard candy to suck on should you feel sick when you are away from home or traveling.

Exercise
Bending and stretching may make pregnancy sickness worse, so ignore your usual exercise program and routine household chores for a while. Fresh air and gentle exercise are often helpful, even if it is only a short walk.

Rest
In these early days of pregnancy it's important to get extra rest, especially if you're suffering from pregnancy sickness. This can be difficult if you have a busy and demanding job, but try to delegate some of your responsibilities. When you're feeling sick, loosen your belt and other tight clothing and take a short break. Try going to bed earlier and giving yourself an additional two or three hours sleep each night.

When Nothing Works
For a few women pregnancy sickness is a constant and continual misery. If you are very ill throughout the day and cannot keep anything down, tell your doctor. There is currently no FDA-approved medication available for acute cases of nausea and vomiting, but many physicians recommend a vitamin B_6 supplement and yeast extract.

Heartburn
In early pregnancy heartburn is probably caused by excess stomach acid being regurgitated into the lower part of the esophagus, the canal that connects the stomach to the mouth. It is this acid that causes a burning sensation around your chest. Heartburn may also occur later in pregnancy.
The eating tips that help alleviate pregnancy sickness also help to

relieve heartburn. Eat several small meals instead of one or two large ones, and wait an hour or so after your last meal before going to bed. Eat slowly and drink plenty of fluids. You might try sleeping propped up with several pillows. Avoid bending and stretching throughout the day.

If all this fails, your physician may recommend an antacid or other form of medication, but don't treat yourself with over-the-counter preparations.

CRAVINGS

Some pregnant women have cravings for, or aversions to, certain smells, foods, or drinks. These may include a sudden dislike for coffee, or a new desire for anchovies. Some crave pickles and sharp-tasting foods, while others want only bland foods or sweets. The cause of these cravings is uncertain, but they probably don't have anything to do with your nutritional needs. You don't crave chocolate bars because your body needs an extra dose of sugar or caffeine.

Cravings may have something to do with hormonal influences on your sense of taste. Eating the foods you crave is all right as long as you don't go to extremes, and as long as you continue to meet your nutritional requirements.

The only time to worry about a craving is if you find yourself unexpectedly yearning to taste a nonfood substance, such as clay or tar. It sounds bizarre but this occasionally does happen to pregnant women. Consumption probably wouldn't kill you, but doctors advise women not to succumb.

Some women get a metallic taste in their mouths in the early part of pregnancy which affects the taste of food, but this usually disappears later.

Symptoms in Fathers-to-Be

Women aren't the only ones to experience the early symptoms of pregnancy. One surprising new study has shown that prospective fathers often have similar symptoms. Michael, one of the expectant fathers studied by researchers at University of Wisconsin-Milwaukee School of Nursing, gained weight, was easily irritated, took afternoon naps, and had excruciating backaches. The day his daughter was born, his symptoms disappeared, he began to lose weight, and he was soon back to his easygoing, energetic self.

This phenomenon, known as couvade (from the French word meaning to brood or hatch), usually includes such symptoms as Michael's, as well as morning sickness, insomnia, depression, stress, and cravings for a particular food. According to the study led by Dr. Jacqueline Clinton, a nurse and research scientist, couvade is common; of the 147 expectant fathers involved in the study, about 90 percent reported multiple couvade symptoms. Insomnia was the symptom most often reported.

Dr. Clinton and other scientists who have observed the phenomenon believe that couvade is a natural way for a father to express a bond of sympathy with the expectant mother, and also a way to establish his paternity. So far, no one has discovered any physiological reason for couvade symptoms.

Men apparently are reluctant to tell anyone about their symptoms. Yet after several months, the symptoms can become tiring and uncomfortable. Unfortunately no one has offered any solutions for men suffering from couvade symptoms.

ALTERING YOUR EXERCISE PROGRAM IN PREGNANCY

Obstetricians usually advise their patients to continue doing whatever exercise they had been doing prior to pregnancy but reducing the intensity or duration of an exercise as pregnancy progresses.

It's a good idea to avoid unusually vigorous or dangerous sports and exercise. Waterskiing and surfing should definitely be avoided. Most physicians also caution against scuba diving during pregnancy because decompression may be potentially hazardous to the fetus. Your center of gravity changes as your abdomen enlarges during pregnancy, so if you ski or ice skate you may have more trouble keeping your balance. Obviously, pregnancy is not a good time to learn either of these sports. However, if you're an accomplished skier or skater, you can continue the sport, but downgrade the difficulty.

The American College of Obstetricians and Gynecologists has recently suggested that aerobic sorts of exercises seem to provide the best all-around exercise program for pregnant women—brisk walking, swimming, and stationary cycling. Whatever exercise you choose, always stop before you are exhausted or any time that you feel pain.

The Pre-Pregnancy Shape-Up exercises described in Chapter 11 can be continued throughout pregnancy.

SEX DURING PREGNANCY

Many couples enjoy a particularly good intimate relationship during pregnancy. However, if you have had one or more miscarriages or a previous premature labor, ask your doctor's advice regarding sexual intercourse in the first trimester.

Although there has been some controversy about the safety of sexual intercourse in the last weeks of pregnancy, most physicians feel that there is no danger unless a woman has a history of childbirth complications. The fetus is well protected by the amniotic fluid, which acts as a cushion against bumps; the mucus plug in the cervix gives added protection. Nor do contractions during a woman's orgasm appear to harm the fetus. The uterus normally contracts regularly throughout a woman's reproductive lifetime, although the contractions are unfelt. The precise effects of orgasm on the fetus are unknown but are considered without hazard. Some obstetricians advise against orgasm during the last three months of pregnancy if a woman has a previous history of premature labor.

Sexual desire seems to fluctuate along a curve during pregnancy. Some women lose interest in sex during the first trimester, especially if they suffer from fatigue or nausea and vomiting. Often sexual desire turns during the second and third trimester, then wanes again toward the end of pregnancy.

Sometimes the cervix becomes fragile and may be slightly damaged during an internal examination or during intercourse, resulting in light spotting. If you notice any bleeding, you should not have intercourse and tell your doctor.

The reason that some doctors advise against intercourse in the last few weeks of pregnancy is that after the mucus plug guarding the neck of the cervix comes away, the membranes surrounding the baby are exposed to potential infection. Your obstetrician will check the condition of the cervix during each internal exam and tell you when the membranes are exposed.

ADJUSTMENTS AT WORK

In the early months of pregnancy, when you may feel sick or fatigued, try to arrange a flexible work schedule so that you can take more time getting up in the morning and travel outside the rush hour. Most pregnant women can expect to feel much better after the third month of pregnancy, although every woman continues to need more sleep and rest throughout pregnancy.

In general, there is no need to stop working until you feel ready, or until your doctor advises you to do so. All pregnant women should avoid strenuous activity, extreme temperatures, smoking areas, and excessive stair climbing. Find a few minutes during the day when you can sit with your feet up. Wearing support hose will help reduce swelling in your ankles and help prevent varicose veins. In the last three months particularly, avoid prolonged standing, heavy lifting, and frequent stooping and bending. If your job involves these tasks, ask for help from colleagues.

If you haven't already done so, discuss with your obstetrician any possible health hazards in your working environment so that he or she can advise you of any precautions that can be taken to protect you and the baby (see Chapter 8).

TRAVEL

Generally, traveling is harmless as far as the fetus is concerned, but there are some ground rules. Sitting in the same position for a long time can affect blood circulation to your legs. Not emptying your bladder for many hours also encourages bladder infections, which are more common during pregnancy. Don't take travel-sickness remedies without consulting your doctor.

If you travel by plane, don't drink alcohol to steady your nerves. If you have a threatening miscarriage in early pregnancy, it is unwise to fly. It is also unwise to fly in a small unpressurized plane because the decrease in oxygen could be harmful to the baby.

Driving a car is safe, provided it does not make you too tired and you do not suffer from dizzy spells. On a long journey, stop every two or so hours to stretch your legs and empty your bladder. Using a seat belt with a shoulder harness is always wise, even in the later stages when you may find the belt uncomfortable.

Altitude Sickness

Anyone can suffer from mountain sickness. Symptoms include headache, nausea, insomnia, vomiting, fatigue, and—in more serious cases—shortness of breath and pneumonialike symptoms. Pregnant women especially should take things easy for a day or two after arrival at a high-altitude location so the body has time to adjust to the lower oxygen pressure and to ensure that the supply of oxygen to the fetus continues smoothly.

Pregnant women visiting high altitudes also need to use good sunscreen, since they are more susceptible to pigmentary changes and there is more solar radiation at high altitudes.

CHOOSING YOUR BABY'S DOCTOR

Every baby needs his or her own doctor. It's a good idea to choose a pediatrician before your baby is born. A pre-baby visit will give both you and your partner an opportunity to talk with the doctor in a relaxed atmosphere. The relationship between the doctor and the parents and child is important and continues for several years. Make your choice as carefully as when you chose your own obstetrician.

Regular examinations are the only way you can be certain that your baby is thriving and developing properly. For these examinations, your baby can visit a baby clinic, your family doctor, or a pediatrician.

Your family doctor or obstetrician can recommend a pediatrician. The names of pediatricians can also be obtained from hospitals and from your local medical society. Information about baby clinics can be obtained at the hospital where your baby was born, from city or county health departments, or from the Visiting Nurse Association.

Consider the same elements: credentials, locations, hospital affiliations, and fees. For pediatricians, there are some less obvious matters to consider: Does the doctor make house calls? How can he or she be reached in an emergency, and how will he or she be covered when unavailable? The nurses and office support staff are also important. When you call, you want to hear a friendly, understanding voice on the telephone.

The most essential factors in choosing a pediatrician are communication and confidence, the feeling that you can discuss the smallest thing with your baby's doctor without feeling that you are being overanxious. The physician you choose should answer all of your questions, including those that concern simply the day-to-day problems of caring for an infant.

One older mother, who brought her newly adopted year-old daughter to a family Thanksgiving dinner, became hysterical when the baby woke up late in the evening and began to cry uncontrollably. Tears poured down the child's cheeks, and the worried mother walked the baby back and forth for half an hour. The mother wanted to call the baby's pediatrician; the father said she was silly and overreacting.

"She ate too much," he said. "She's not used to so many people. There's nothing wrong with her."

"But what if she's really sick?" asked the mother. "How can we know for sure?"

A quarrel erupted between the parents, and the frantic mother dialed the pediatrician's home number. At nine-thirty on Thanksgiving night the doctor came on the line, calmed the mother's anxiety, spoke to the angry father, suggested that they give the baby some apple juice and take her home. If she hadn't quieted down after they got home, they were to call the doctor back at once. In this case, the pediatrician was as much marriage counselor as she was physician. For first-time parents, that kind of pediatrician is an invaluable ally.

When the Pediatrician Comes on the Scene
The pediatrician you choose will examine the baby on the first day of birth and just before the baby leaves the hospital. After that he or she will probably want to see the baby once a month for at least the first four to six months.

At these regular visits the doctor will weigh and measure and thoroughly examine the baby for all the signs that indicate normal development. Your baby will also receive a series of inoculations according to a schedule based on worldwide experience in the protection of children.

The most successful parent-pediatrician relationships are full-fledged partnerships to which both sides bring something of value. The pediatrician knows what is within a normal range of behavior, but only you will know what is normal for your child. The information you offer the pediatrician is crucial to his or her providing excellent medical care for your child.

EMOTIONAL IMPACT

When you first learn you are going to have a baby your emotions may be mixed. Every change generates some emotional upheaval and one of life's biggest changes is adding a baby to your life. Even the most eagerly anticipated pregnancy brings some conflicts and worries, sometimes exaggerated because of mood swings during the first trimester of pregnancy. Both partners may experience several different emotions, ranging from delight to sheer terror. And all of these emotions may be equally felt, perhaps all at the same time.

When a woman feels ill and tired at the beginning of pregnancy the picture may seem bleak indeed. The feelings you worked out before pregnancy may have some residual impact—worries you thought you had resolved may be renewed, and that old familiar ambivalence may return. The anticipated pleasures of parenthood may be dampened by anxiety over the responsibility it entails, as your intellectual and emotional decision to have a baby has become flesh and blood.

Just because you resolved your doubts earlier doesn't mean that you can't talk about them again. Some issues have to be solved many times before they settle down and become familiar and comfortable. Usually talk, time, and adjustments—both physical and emotional—make your doubts disappear.

If you are happy about your pregnancy, you want to shout the news from the rooftops and then dash out to buy maternity clothes. Or you may want to keep the news to yourselves for a while. If you still feel ambivalent about pregnancy, or if you have suffered previous miscarriages, you may want to wait awhile before telling anyone. When, how, and whom to tell is a personal decision.

Each partner is the other's greatest ally as you embark on this unique adventure. Millions of human beings have shared a similar experience, but this one is yours alone and in the history of the world there will never be another one like it.

Millions of years of instinct have not prepared prospective parents for modern society. Life today is not simple. Rearing a child to thrive in an increasingly complex world is an increasingly complex job. Pre-pregnancy planning is a new concept that fills the gap between our instinctive desire to have children and the reality of bringing children into this high-tech, fast-paced, mercurial society. Medical technologies are multiplying so fast that it's crucial to become knowledgeable ahead of time if you want to make the right decisions and have the best choices available to you when you become pregnant. Preparation means that you can gain the maximum benefits from technology and still give your children all of the love and attention they need within the bosom of a stable family.

The medical establishment is just now beginning to recognize that pre-pregnancy fitness is an important health issue. *Self* magazine reports that John T. Queenan, M.D., a professor and chairman of the Obstetrics and Gynecology Department at Georgetown University Medical Center designed a class called Preparation for Pregnancy offered for nonpregnant students. At the Omega Institutes, a new high-tech woman's hospital in New Orleans, seminars are offered in pre-pregnancy planning. In New York several well-known obstetricians are routinely offering pre-pregnancy medical examination. These scientists predict that pre-pregnancy planning will become standard in the future—and when you read this book you become a pioneer in a growing trend born from a very real modern need.

Choosing to have children today means understanding the promises of parenthood and being physically and emotionally prepared before conception. By taking an overview of your circumstances and the world into which you will bring your child, you will be able to enjoy pregnancy more, and at the same time create a more stable and relaxed environment for your entire family. By following a program of pre-pregnancy preparation you are acting to ensure the best future for your child.

Pre-pregnancy planning also means that in a society overwhelmed by technology you don't have to compromise the traditional values of pregnancy and childbirth. It offers a way to preserve all the best parts of parenting—the warmth and regeneration of family life.

If you choose to have a child, your commitment demands an investment of time and learning, as well as love. Preparation and plan-

258 THE PRE-PREGNANCY PLANNER

ning should begin the moment you make the parenthood decision. And this investment will pay all the dividends for a happy and healthy pregnancy and a more fulfilling family experience—dividends that will last a lifetime.

INDEX

chronic, 205
ectopic pregnancy and, 195
infertility and, 203–4
Environmental effects on
  pregnancy, 70–87, 147–48
  alcohol, 72–74
  altitude, 80
  birth defects, 153, 155
  caffeine, 74–75
  diet and, 106
  drugs, 75–78
  fetal alcohol syndrome, 73
  heat, 79–80
  industrial waste, 82–83
  infertility and, 206
  male reproductive system and,
    75, 77–78
  miscarriage and, 193
  occupational. See Occupational
    hazards to pregnancy
  pollution, 78, 82–83
  radiation, 84, 85
  rubella, 145, 155
  smoking, 70–72
  stress, 78–79
  teratogens, 82
Episiotomy: exercise and, 130–31
Exercise(s), 130–41, 147
  for abdominal muscles, 136–38
  to avoid, 131–32
  for back muscles, 138–41
  diet and, 113
  episiotomy and, 130–31
  general, 131–32
  goal of, 130–31
  infertility and, 132
  late pregnancy and, 190
  for pelvic floor muscles, 134–36
  during pregnancy, 251–52
  pregnancy sickness and, 249
  Pre-Pregnancy Shape Up, 134–41
  specific, 132–33
  vitamins and, 113

Fallopian tubes, 62
  chlamydia and, 91

infertility and, 203–4
silicone implants in, 102–3
Families
  dual career, 24, 26, 29–32, 39
  female-headed, 19
  men in, 18
  sense of, 15
  seven stages of, 14–15
  shapes of, 17
  single-parent, 3, 19–20
  spacing of babies in, 23
  step-, 20–21
  traditional, 17–18
  See also Parenthood
Family-centered maternity care,
  236–37
Family day homes, 44
Fatherhood (fathers)
  careers and, 26–27, 29–32
  See also Men; Parenthood
Fats and oils, 117
FDA Consumer (magazine), 76
Female reproductive system, 62
  cervix, 62, 196–97, 205
  chlamydia and, 88, 90–93
  pelvic inflammatory disease and,
    88–91, 94, 96, 97, 202, 203
  scarring of. See Pelvic
    inflammatory disease (PID)
  uterus, 62, 67
  vagina, 62
  See also Fertility; Infertility
Fertility, 66–69
  age and, 12, 186
  enhancement of, 214–27
  hypothalamus and, 207
  menstrual cycle and, 67
  pelvic inflammatory disease and,
    89–90
  predicting, 68–69
  protecting, 88–104
  tests for, timing of, 212
  See also Infertility
Fertility specialists, 211
Fertility workup, 211, 212
Fetal alcohol syndrome, 73

Printed in the United States
by Baker & Taylor Publisher Services